Mindfulness for Pain Management

A Holistic Approach to Healing Chronic Pain, Reducing Stress, and Cultivating Emotional Resilience

Dr. Marie Josée Benoit md

Pierre Beaulnes

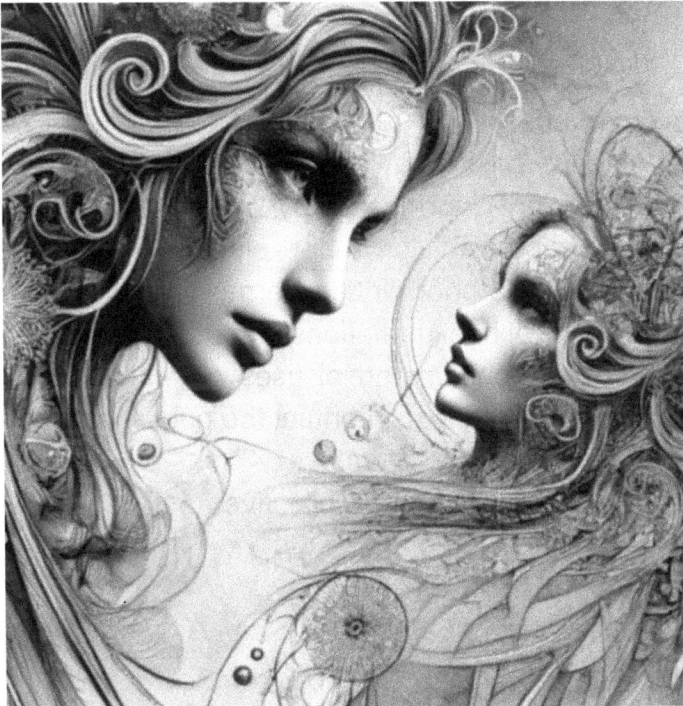

Ætherial Dreams Collective

"Empowering Minds, Enlightening Souls"

Published by Ætherial Dreams Collective
Vancouver, British Columbia
ISBN: 979-8-89587-911-5
First Edition: February 2025
Printed in Canada

Table of Contents

4

Introduction

Imagine waking up every morning, your mind already bracing for the familiar tide of pain that greets you with the day. For over 50 million adults in the U.S., this scenario is not merely a hypothetical—it's a reality. Chronic pain, like an uninvited guest, lingers long after its initial appearance, affecting daily life and overshadowing precious moments. To those experiencing it, chronic pain can feel like living under an endless cloud, dimming the vibrancy of life's experiences. Yet, what if there existed a way to transform this relationship with pain, allowing for pockets of peace and happiness amidst the struggle?

Welcome to "Mindfulness for Pain Management: A Holistic Approach to Healing Chronic Pain, Reducing Stress, and Cultivating Emotional Resilience." This book offers more than just temporary relief; it invites you on a journey toward reclaiming control of your life through mindfulness, a practice rooted in awareness and tranquility. Here, we delve into practical techniques designed to seamlessly integrate into your daily routine, offering you the tools to lessen pain perception and elevate your quality of life.

This guidebook is about turning theory into practice, translating abstract concepts into tangible steps that empower you in managing not only your physical discomfort but also the emotional toll that often accompanies chronic pain. Through actionable strategies grounded in scientific research, you'll discover how mindfulness acts as a transformative agent in pain management, enhancing both mental fortitude and emotional well-being.

Let us consider the unique benefits mindfulness brings to the table. Instead of viewing pain as an adversary to be battled, mindfulness encourages a relationship based on understanding and acceptance. By cultivating presence in each moment, you learn to navigate pain without being overwhelmed by it. It's akin to taming a wild beast—not eradicating its existence, but coexisting with compassion and resilience. Picture yourself riding atop the waves of pain rather than being swallowed beneath them. Mindfulness empowers you to pivot from simply surviving to truly thriving, even amidst adversity.

How does this transformation unfold? With step-by-step practices detailed in our chapters, tailored to various pain conditions, you will be equipped to reshape your experience of pain. These methods are not meant to replace traditional medical treatments but to complement them, creating a balanced approach to health and healing. As you progress through this book, pay attention to stories shared by individuals who have walked similar paths. Their narratives may echo your own struggles, providing insights and encouragement to bolster your efforts.

The journey through this book promises positivity and achievable growth. Rather than perceiving chronic pain as a solitary, lifelong sentence, consider the possibility of connection—with yourself, your body, and the world around you. This curated collection of wisdom and relatable real-life tales aims to act as a trustworthy companion during times of uncertainty. With each chapter, you will unlock new layers of understanding and capabilities, bringing you closer to embracing the entirety of your being.

As a reader, you may find yourself asking vital questions: How can practicing mindfulness specifically alleviate chronic pain? What tangible techniques can be implemented to yield stress reduction and foster emotional resilience? And importantly, how does strengthening emotional resilience impact one's overall experience of pain? Throughout these pages, you'll uncover answers grounded in evidence and empathy, equipping you to face everyday challenges with renewed confidence.

In our fast-paced world, the pursuit of instant solutions often overshadows slower, introspective approaches. However, the path illuminated by mindfulness requires patience and commitment. It encourages stepping back, taking a breath, and observing the fuller picture of your lived experience. It's an invitation to explore profound shifts in perspective that open doors to inner peace, even when outward circumstances remain unchanged.

For caregivers and family members supporting loved ones with chronic pain, this book offers insight into providing meaningful assistance while navigating your own emotional complexities. Meanwhile, health and wellness professionals will find valuable knowledge and techniques to enhance their practice, enabling better support for their clients' journeys toward holistic pain management.

At its heart, "Mindfulness for Pain Management" is about hope—hope that lies within reach, encouraging every individual grappling with ongoing pain to seek brighter horizons. Embrace this opportunity to transform your life through mindful engagement, where empowerment arises from understanding, acceptance, and sustained action.

So, are you ready to embark on this transformative journey? As you turn these pages, know that each word is a step toward reshaping your relationship with pain. The final destination may differ for everyone, but the promise remains the same—a more profound connection with the self, greater resilience, and the rekindled ability to find joy amidst life's challenges.

In the words ahead, embrace curiosity and openness. Allow mindfulness to reveal not only the depths of your strength but also the heights of potential flourishing, crafting a narrative of healing uniquely your own. Welcome to a new chapter, where the power to manage pain and nurture emotional resilience is at your fingertips.

CHAPTER 1

Understanding Chronic Pain
and Mindfulness

Understanding chronic pain and mindfulness can seem like navigating a complex web of sensations, emotions, and responses that weave through our daily lives. Chronic pain, which lasts longer than three months, becomes an unwelcome companion that affects every facet of life—physically, emotionally, and socially. The journey to managing this persistent discomfort is not merely about enduring; it's about finding new paths to coexist with, and ideally, alleviate the burden it imposes. Here, mindfulness emerges as a beacon of hope, offering a transformative approach to dealing with the intricate layers of chronic pain. It guides us gently toward acceptance and awareness, providing tools to observe our experiences without judgment, transforming how we relate to our pain.

In this chapter, we'll delve into the nature of chronic pain, exploring its varied forms and impacts on those who live with it daily. We'll uncover the misconceptions and stigma surrounding this invisible condition, recognizing how these societal narratives influence not just public understanding but also personal experience. Moreover, we'll introduce mindfulness as a method for managing chronic pain, focusing on how its principles can help shift perceptions and responses to pain. By examining the scientific foundations supporting mindfulness techniques, we aim to provide insights that empower you to manage your pain more effectively. This exploration will unfold potential pathways to enhance your quality of life, fostering resilience and self-compassion along the way.

Definition and Types of Chronic Pain

Chronic pain is an intricate condition that affects millions of people worldwide. Defined as pain lasting longer than three months, it significantly impacts both physical and mental well-being (Katz et al., 2015). Unlike acute pain, which serves as the body's warning signal, chronic pain persists without purpose, leading to a cascade of challenges in daily life. It can become all-consuming, affecting individuals' ability to perform even the simplest of daily tasks, from getting out of bed in the morning to maintaining employment. This persistence of pain often causes distress and suffering, altering one's overall quality of life.

Misunderstanding surrounding chronic pain adds another layer of difficulty for those who endure it. Many people may mistakenly believe that if there is no visible cause or injury, the pain must not be real or significant. This misconception perpetuates stigma and isolation, leaving patients to suffer silently. They may feel disbelieved and alone, as chronic pain conditions often lack straightforward explanations (Cohen et al., 2022). Consequently, these individuals find themselves trapped within their own bodies, experiencing not only physical discomfort but also emotional and social detachment.

One crucial aspect to grasp about chronic pain is the diversity within its types, each requiring tailored relief strategies. Nociceptive pain, for example, originates from tissue damage or inflammation and typically responds well to conventional pain medications and therapies. Neuropathic pain, resulting from nerve damage, might necessitate treatments such as anti-seizure medications or antidepressants that alter how the nervous system processes pain signals. Psychogenic pain, though less understood, is linked to psychological factors but is no less real for those who experience it. Each type of pain presents unique challenges in management and requires specific approaches to find effective relief (Katz et al., 2015).

Raising awareness about various pain conditions plays a pivotal role in promoting empathy and understanding for those affected. Chronic pain is not just an extended version of acute pain; it is a complex interplay between physical, emotional, and sometimes psychological factors. By fostering greater comprehension, society can begin to dismantle the barriers of stigma and disbelief that so many with chronic pain encounter. Education and open conversations can help create an environment where individuals living with chronic pain feel supported and validated.

Moreover, recognizing the ripple effects of chronic pain on a person's life, relationships, and activities can lead to more comprehensive approaches in addressing it. For instance, acknowledging the emotional toll it takes can encourage healthcare providers to incorporate mental health support into treatment plans. Patients battling chronic pain often face anxiety, depression, and a general sense of helplessness, which can exacerbate their symptoms. Addressing these mental health components through therapy or counseling can improve pain management outcomes and enhance the overall quality of life.

Understanding and accepting the reality of chronic pain can also extend into the workplace and community settings. Employers can play a vital role by accommodating employees with chronic pain, implementing flexible work arrangements or modifying job responsibilities when possible. This not only aids in reducing absenteeism and enhancing productivity but also sends a powerful message of inclusivity and understanding.

Empathy towards those experiencing chronic pain involves seeing beyond the immediate symptoms and recognizing the broader implications. It requires viewing each person holistically, considering the myriad of ways chronic pain intertwines with their daily existence. Whether it's a parent striving to participate in their child's activities, an athlete adjusting to new limitations, or an older adult adapting to increased dependence, chronic pain reshapes lives in profound ways.

In the journey toward improving chronic pain management, it is essential to shift perspectives—moving from questioning the validity of someone's pain to understanding its complexities and offering genuine support. By increasing public awareness and encouraging open dialogues, society can break down misconceptions and stigma surrounding chronic pain. In doing so, we move closer to a world where those affected can live with dignity, respect, and improved quality of life, knowing they are not alone in their experience.

Impact of Chronic Pain on Quality of Life

Living with chronic pain often feels like navigating a never-ending storm. Its impacts stretch far beyond the physical boundaries of one's body, seeping into emotional well-being and social interactions, leaving enduring marks on living standards and happiness. For many, chronic pain becomes a shadow that dims life satisfaction and joy. The persistent discomfort can make simple pleasures unbearable, pulling individuals away from activities they once loved and driving them toward isolation.

With every activity constrained by pain, the enthusiasm for life diminishes, turning vibrant experiences into burdens.

The emotional toll is equally profound. Chronic pain has a deceptive way of isolating its sufferers, creating barriers between them and their surroundings. As the days blend into months and then years, the cumulative frustration and helplessness can lead to heightened feelings of anxiety and depression. Emotional distress becomes a companion, exacerbated by the perception that others might not fully comprehend the magnitude of one's daily struggles. Social relationships suffer as a result, causing further withdrawal. Friends and family may find it challenging to engage as they had before, either due to sympathy fatigue or misunderstanding the depth of suffering involved. Over time, this loss of connection contributes to an ever-evolving cycle of loneliness.

Yet, acknowledging these effects is crucial in steering towards a path of comprehensive healing. It's about recognizing that chronic pain isn't just a physical ailment; it's an intricate web of sensory, cognitive, and interpersonal challenges that require more than just medical treatment. This realization propels us toward adopting holistic approaches to healing, aiming to mend not only the body but also the mind and spirit.

Addressing the multifaceted nature of chronic pain is pivotal in promoting effective management. A holistic approach involves looking at pain from numerous vantage points— physically, psychologically, and socially. For instance, integrating psychological support can help mitigate the emotional distress that intertwines with physical pain. Therapies such as cognitive behavioral therapy (CBT) and acceptance and commitment therapy (ACT) have shown promise in helping individuals develop coping strategies, altering how pain is perceived and experienced.

Social support plays a vital role in managing chronic pain holistically. Surrounding oneself with a supportive network can significantly buffer emotional distress. Research indicates that individuals with robust social networks often report lower levels of pain severity and disability. Group-based interventions become powerful tools within this framework, fostering a sense of community and belonging among those who understand each other's struggles intimately. Through shared experiences within these groups, individuals can rediscover a sense of agency and hope, breaking the cycle of isolation.

Moreover, addressing chronic pain through education can empower patients and their families. Understanding the biopsychosocial model of pain helps in appreciating that pain is not merely a physiological response but an interplay of diverse factors. Education can dispel myths surrounding chronic pain, reducing stigma and encouraging more open conversations about its challenges and realities.

Incorporating mindfulness practices offers another dimension to holistic management. Mindfulness trains individuals to focus on the present moment, cultivating awareness, acceptance, and self-compassion. Engaging in mindfulness techniques, such as mindful breathing or meditation, provides tools to navigate pain without judgment, altering the emotional response to discomfort. Thus, while mindfulness does not necessarily eliminate pain, it transforms the experience of it, providing mental resilience and bolstering emotional health.

Physical therapies should also align with a holistic approach. Movement and exercise, tailored to individual capacities, not only enhance physical function but also elevate mood and social engagement. By integrating physical activity into one's routine in a gentle, sustainable manner, individuals can reclaim aspects of their lives previously overshadowed by pain.

Healthcare systems must also evolve to adopt this holistic perspective, shifting towards models that prioritize collaborative care. Encouraging interdisciplinary teams—consisting of doctors, therapists, nutritionists, and more—ensures that various facets of a patient's life are considered in treatment plans. This multidisciplinary approach fosters comprehensive improvements, particularly in familial and social contexts, where support and understanding can dramatically influence outcomes.

Overall, comprehending the pervasive reach of chronic pain is the first step toward mastering its management. While it may seem daunting, the journey toward more satisfying and joyful living begins with a shift in perspective. Recognizing and addressing the broader impacts of pain—emotional, social, and physical—is instrumental in crafting a life that thrives despite ongoing challenges. Healing, therefore, becomes not merely about reducing symptoms but about enhancing quality of life through empathy, understanding, and connectivity.

Introduction to Mindfulness for Pain Management

Mindfulness, at its core, is a practice of focused awareness on the present moment. It's about shifting our attention deliberately to our current experiences without judgment or distraction. By embracing this approach, individuals can cultivate self-compassion and acceptance, which are crucial for managing chronic pain effectively.

The principles of mindfulness—attention, acceptance, and intention—are foundational in establishing realistic expectations when dealing with pain. These elements teach us to pay close attention to what we are experiencing right now, whether it's physical discomfort or emotional stress. Acceptance involves acknowledging these sensations without resistance, avoiding the common tendency to fight against them or deny their presence. Intention directs us towards choosing how we wish to engage with our experiences, allowing for a more conscious and compassionate response to pain.

A simple yet powerful technique within mindfulness is focused breathing. This practice involves bringing awareness to your breath, noticing each inhalation and exhalation, and the sensations associated with this natural rhythm. When chronic pain strikes, focused breathing serves as an anchor, drawing attention away from distress and reducing stress levels. It helps in calming the mind and easing tension in the body, thus playing a crucial role in pain management.

While mindfulness might not eliminate pain completely, it transforms the experience of pain by altering how we perceive it. Through regular practice, individuals learn to observe their pain without becoming overwhelmed by it. This shift in perspective empowers them to build resilience, making them less reactive to the peaks and troughs of their condition. Over time, the mindful approach fosters an environment where pain does not define one's ability to live a fulfilling life.

Kirsten Neff, renowned for her work on self-compassion, highlights how mindfulness changes the brain's response to pain. By encouraging relaxation, mindfulness reduces cortisol levels—a stress hormone linked to chronic pain (Shlafman, 2023). Thus, the practice not only aids immediate coping but also contributes to long-term well-being.

Another essential aspect of mindfulness is developing self-compassion. In accepting that pain is part of the human experience, individuals can treat themselves with the same kindness and understanding they would offer to others facing similar struggles. This element of mindfulness involves nurturing oneself in moments of difficulty, breaking free from cycles of frustration and helplessness that often accompany chronic pain (Mead, 2019).

Practicing self-compassion through mindfulness helps individuals redirect negative thoughts associated with pain, such as blaming oneself or feeling inadequate. This transformation from self-criticism to self-care bolsters psychological resilience and promotes healing. Building a mindful self-compassion practice begins with identifying personal barriers to self-kindness and replacing them with supportive beliefs.

Moreover, mindfulness encourages non-judgmental awareness, which is pivotal in chronic pain management. By observing pain without labeling it as 'bad' or 'unbearable,' individuals can lessen its emotional impact. This change in mindset enables a more measured response to pain stimuli, enhancing one's ability to cope effectively (Shlafman, 2023).

Empirical studies confirm mindfulness's efficacy in alleviating chronic pain symptoms. For instance, research has demonstrated that mindfulness-based interventions can significantly reduce the perception of pain, even if the physiological sensation remains unchanged. Participants report not only reduced pain intensity but also improved mood and overall quality of life following mindfulness training.

Mindfulness instills a greater sense of control over one's body and mind, empowering those with chronic pain to navigate their daily lives more comfortably. As individuals become adept at maintaining present-moment awareness, they develop a deeper understanding of their body's signals, allowing for timely and appropriate responses to pain episodes.

Ultimately, mindfulness offers a compassionate pathway to living alongside chronic pain. It encourages a harmonious relationship between mind and body, fostering an environment where acceptance and resilience flourish. By integrating mindfulness into their daily routine, individuals can reclaim a sense of peace, despite the challenges posed by their condition.

History and Integration of Mindfulness in Healthcare

Mindfulness has deep roots in ancient Eastern philosophies, originating from Buddhist and Hindu traditions where practices like meditation were central to spiritual development. These teachings emphasized the importance of being fully present, cultivating awareness, and understanding the nature of human suffering. Today, these foundational principles inform the modern adaptation of mindfulness within healthcare as a vital component for managing chronic pain.

At the forefront of this integration is Mindfulness-Based Stress Reduction (MBSR), developed by Jon Kabat-Zinn in the late 1970s. MBSR is a structured program that offers clear, systematic methodologies for incorporating mindfulness into daily life, specifically designed to address stress and enhance well-being. It involves a combination of meditation, yoga, and body-awareness exercises, providing practitioners with tools to manage stress and pain more effectively (Kriakous et al., 2021).

The methodology's simplicity and efficacy have contributed to its widespread adoption in medical settings.

Incorporating mindfulness into healthcare represents a broader shift toward holistic care, where treating the whole person—mind, body, and spirit—is prioritized over merely addressing symptoms. This approach recognizes that emotional and psychological well-being are integral to physical health. Research shows remarkable improvements in patient outcomes when mindfulness practices are integrated into treatment plans. Patients often report reduced stress, improved mood, and decreased reliance on medication, reflecting the benefits of a more comprehensive treatment strategy (Srour & Keyes, 2024).

The growing acceptance of mindfulness within medical contexts is bolstered by substantial research supporting its effectiveness. Numerous studies document how mindfulness can alter neurological pathways, enhancing an individual's ability to cope with pain and stress. The increase in scholarly attention has led to refined techniques and evidence-based applications that underscore mindfulness as a credible and reliable form of intervention. For instance, studies conducted by Chiesa and Serretti (2009) demonstrate mindfulness's role in reducing anxiety and boosting self-compassion among participants, further proving its viability.

One significant aspect of mindfulness in healthcare is its focus on empowering patients through active participation in their healing process. By encouraging individuals to engage with their own experiences non-judgmentally, mindfulness fosters a proactive stance toward health management. Patients learn to observe their thoughts and emotions with greater clarity, resulting in improved self-regulation and adaptive coping mechanisms (Shapiro et al., 2006). As a result, individuals become more adept at handling the emotional complexities of living with chronic pain, ultimately improving their quality of life.

Complementary practices between mindfulness and conventional medical treatments offer a comprehensive strategy for addressing chronic conditions. The capacity of mindfulness-based interventions to work alongside pharmacological therapies presents a multimodal approach to pain relief. By engaging central brain networks involved in pain regulation, mindfulness provides an alternative path for patients wary of medication dependence or side effects associated with long-term pharmaceutical use. This synergy opens the door to transformative health care approaches, where personalization and patient empowerment are central (Kriakous et al., 2021).

To illustrate its impact, consider the scenario where patients suffering from conditions like fibromyalgia or chronic headaches participate in mindfulness programs. Studies indicate significant reductions in perceived pain severity and an improvement in overall functional capacity when mindfulness is incorporated into treatment regimens. Participants often experience enhanced emotional resilience, a sense of community, and increased motivation to engage in self-care practices. This highlights mindfulness as not just a temporary relief mechanism but as a sustainable lifestyle change that supports both mental and physical health (Srour & Keyes, 2024).

Healthcare providers play a crucial role in facilitating the integration of mindfulness into patient care. By embracing mindfulness themselves, clinicians can model presence, empathy, and nonjudgmental communication, fostering stronger patient-provider relationships. This engagement encourages patients to explore mindfulness as a viable treatment option, knowing they have support from their medical team.

Despite its growing popularity, accessibility remains a challenge. Patients may be unfamiliar with mindfulness or skeptical of its benefits compared to traditional treatments. Educating patients about the physiological processes underlying pain and mindfulness's role in modulating these processes can bridge this gap. Health professionals should ensure access to resources, whether through local classes, online courses, or reputable self-help materials, to empower patients in their journey toward mindfulness (Kriakous et al., 2021).

Mindfulness and Its Scientific Foundations

Mindfulness has emerged as a transformative approach in managing chronic pain, supported by scientific principles and research highlighting its benefits. At its core, mindfulness engages cognitive and emotional processes, reshaping how pain is perceived. This practice emphasizes present-moment awareness, allowing individuals to focus on the current experience without judgment. By doing so, mindfulness helps to reduce the emotional distress associated with pain, offering relief beyond conventional pain management techniques (Zeidan & Vago, 2016).

The cognitive shift facilitated by mindfulness can significantly influence pain perception. Chronic pain often comes with negative emotions and stress, which can exacerbate the pain experience. Mindfulness helps cultivate an open-minded acceptance, reducing emotional reactivity and promoting self-compassion. This change in mindset can diminish the severity of pain experienced, as individuals learn to decouple the sensory aspect of pain from the emotional responses it elicits (Sodeman,

2020). By fostering an attitude of acceptance towards pain, individuals may find that their overall sense of suffering decreases.

Physiologically, mindfulness practices have been shown to alter brain activity in ways beneficial for pain management. Studies using neuroimaging technologies have identified specific brain areas affected by mindfulness meditation, such as the anterior cingulate cortex and insula. These regions are involved in modulating pain response, suggesting that mindfulness can enhance top-down control over pain signals (Zeidan & Vago, 2016). This provides a neurological basis for the efficacy of mindfulness in alleviating chronic pain. By engaging these brain networks, mindfulness meditation can help reduce the intensity of pain signals, making them more manageable.

Empirical research continues to support mindfulness as a viable method for pain management. Numerous studies document significant reductions in pain levels and improvements in quality of life among participants engaging in regular mindfulness practice. For example, research conducted by Fadel Zeidan and colleagues revealed that mindfulness training led to less activation in brain areas associated with processing pain messages, showing clear physiological changes related to reduced pain perception (Sodeman, 2020). This growing body of evidence underscores the potential of mindfulness as a non-invasive, cost-effective strategy for managing chronic pain, especially in scenarios where traditional treatments might fall short.

One of the most promising aspects of mindfulness in pain management is its ability to foster long-term emotional resilience and independence. Regular mindfulness practice helps patients develop coping strategies that extend beyond immediate pain relief. These strategies include cultivating patience, nurturing positive thoughts, and enhancing emotional regulation, all of which contribute to a more resilient mental state. Over time, patients can become less reliant on external pain relief methods, gaining confidence in their ability to manage pain through self-regulation and mindfulness techniques.

Importantly, mindfulness not only addresses the physical aspects of pain but also targets the psychological burdens that accompany chronic conditions. By teaching individuals to focus on the present moment, mindfulness reduces rumination about past pain or anxiety about future discomfort. This present-focused awareness can alleviate symptoms of depression and anxiety, common co-morbidities in those suffering from chronic pain (Sodeman, 2020). Through consistent practice, mindfulness helps break the cycle of pain-related stress, fostering a healthier overall mental state.

Patients who embrace mindfulness report feeling more empowered in their pain management journey. This empowerment stems from a newfound sense of control over one's thoughts and emotions. Instead of viewing pain as an insurmountable adversary, individuals learn to coexist with it, acknowledging its presence without being overwhelmed. This shift in perspective can be incredibly liberating, encouraging patients to engage more fully with life and participate in activities they might otherwise avoid due to pain fears.

Ultimately, the integration of mindfulness into chronic pain management represents a holistic approach that respects the complex interplay between mind and body. As more healthcare practitioners recognize the benefits of mindfulness, it may become a staple of comprehensive pain management programs. Its accessibility and adaptability make it an appealing option for those seeking alternative methods to improve their quality of life.

Final Insights

In exploring the intricate nature of chronic pain and how mindfulness can serve as a supportive management tool, we've delved into the varied dimensions that make pain such a complex condition. Pain is not merely a sensation but an experience encompassing physical discomfort, emotional turmoil, and social withdrawal. By understanding this complexity, individuals can begin to reframe their relationship with pain, seeing it not as a solitary battle but a shared journey towards acceptance and resilience. Mindfulness offers a compassionate lens through which to view pain, embracing the present moment with awareness and intention rather than resistance. This empathetic approach empowers individuals to navigate their pain with greater ease, fostering mental well-being alongside physical relief.

As we conclude our exploration of chronic pain and mindfulness, it's important to remember that change begins with small steps. Through practices like mindful breathing and self-compassion, those living with chronic conditions can cultivate a sense of peace amidst their challenges. By not only acknowledging but also accepting one's pain, the path to healing becomes clearer, leading to improved quality of life. The journey may be long and filled with obstacles, but with mindfulness as a trusted companion, each individual can learn to live more fully despite the shadows pain casts. Embrace this mindful journey, and you might find that while pain remains a part of your life, it no longer defines it.

Reference List

Cohen, S. P., Wang, E. J., Doshi, T. L., Vase, L., Cawcutt, K. A., & Tontisirin, N. (2022, March). *Chronic pain and infection: mechanisms, causes, conditions, treatments, and controversies.* BMJ Medicine. https://doi.org/10.1136/bmjmed-2021-000108

Duenas, M., Ojeda, B., Salazar, A., Mico, J. A., & Failde, I. (2016, June). *A review of chronic pain impact on patients, their social environment and the health care system.* Journal of Pain Research. https://doi.org/10.2147/JPR.S105892

Franqueiro, A. R., Yoon, J., Crago, M. A., Curiel, M., & Wilson, J. M. (2023, October 27). *The Interconnection Between Social Support and Emotional Distress Among Individuals with Chronic Pain: A Narrative Review.* Psychology Research and Behavior Management. https://doi.org/10.2147/PRBM.S410606

Kriakous, S. A., Elliott, K. A., Lamers, C., & Owen, R. (2021, September 24). *The effectiveness of mindfulness-based stress reduction on the psychological functioning of healthcare professionals: A systematic review.* Mindfulness. https://doi.org/10.1007/s12671-020-01500-9

Katz, J., Rosenbloom, B. N., & Fashler, S. (2015, April). *Chronic Pain, Psychopathology, and DSM-5 Somatic Symptom Disorder.* The Canadian Journal of Psychiatry. https://doi.org/10.1177/070674371506000402

Mead, E. (2019, June). *What is Mindful Self-Compassion? (Incl. Exercises + Workbooks).* PositivePsychology.com. https://positivepsychology.com/mindful-self-compassion/

Srour, R. A., & Keyes, D. (2024). *Lifestyle Mindfulness In Clinical Practice*. PubMed; StatPearls Publishing. https://www.ncbi.nlm.nih.gov/books/NBK599498/

Sodeman, L. (2020, September 25). *Use mindfulness to cope with chronic pain*. Www.mayoclinichealthsystem.org. https://www.mayoclinichealthsystem.org/hometown-health/speaking-of-health/use-mindfulness-to-cope-with-chronic-pain

Shlafman, M. (2023, June 2). *Origins Holistic Psychotherapy | Dr. Michelle Shlafman LPC, ACS*. Origins Holistic Psychotherapy | Dr. Michelle Shlafman LPC, ACS. https://michelleshlafman.com/blog/empowering-yourself-to-heal-mindfulness-and-self-compassion-for-chronic-pain

Zeidan, F., & Vago, D. R. (2016, June). *Mindfulness meditation-based pain relief: a mechanistic account*. Annals of the New York Academy of Sciences. https://doi.org/10.1111/nyas.13153

CHAPTER 2

The Science Behind Mindfulness

Mindfulness practices have emerged as a beacon of hope for those managing chronic pain, offering a gentle yet powerful approach to well-being. By focusing on the present and encouraging acceptance, mindfulness helps individuals navigate their pain in a way that transcends conventional coping mechanisms. It invites practitioners to observe their thoughts and feelings with curiosity rather than judgment, fostering a sense of inner peace and resilience. This empathetic embrace of one's experience can significantly alter the relationship with pain, transforming it from an adversary into a more approachable aspect of life. The practice acts as a bridge between the mind and body, harmonizing both aspects to reduce stress and promote healing.

In this chapter, we delve into the fascinating science behind mindfulness and its role in pain management. Readers will explore how mindfulness influences brain function, enhancing areas responsible for decision-making and emotional regulation. We'll uncover the neural pathways that mindfulness strengthens, revealing its capacity to modulate the perception of pain and foster resilience. Additionally, the chapter will illuminate the impact of mindfulness on neurotransmitters that promote well-being, painting a comprehensive picture of why these practices are so effective. Through scientific research and insights, we aim to deepen understanding and inspire those seeking alternative methods to regain control over their lives.

Neuroscience of Mindfulness

Mindfulness practices have been increasingly recognized for their profound impact on brain function, particularly in managing pain. A critical element of this process is the activation of specific brain regions like the prefrontal cortex. This area plays a vital role in enhancing decision-making and emotional regulation, both of which are crucial when facing chronic pain. When the prefrontal cortex is engaged through mindfulness practices, individuals often find themselves better equipped to make thoughtful decisions rather than impulsive ones. This can lead to more effective strategies for dealing with pain, such as choosing physical therapy over additional medication (Calderone et al., 2024).

Moreover, mindfulness enhances connectivity in brain areas associated with pain regulation, contributing to structural brain changes over time. Studies have shown that regular mindfulness practice strengthens the connections between regions like the orbitofrontal cortex and the anterior cingulate cortex (ACC). These connections help modulate pain perception and improve the overall processing of painful stimuli (Zeidan et al., 2019). Over time, these changes can alter how an individual experiences pain, potentially leading to significant relief without relying solely on pharmaceutical interventions.

An essential aspect of mindfulness's influence on the brain is its ability to affect neurotransmitter levels. Mindfulness practices have been linked to increased production of serotonin and dopamine, two neurotransmitters known for promoting well-being and motivation. Serotonin acts as a mood stabilizer, often leading to feelings of happiness and calmness, while dopamine is involved in reward and pleasure systems. Together, these neurotransmitters can create a positive feedback loop where engagement in mindfulness activities increases feelings of contentment and motivation, making it easier for individuals to continue the practice, thus fostering greater resilience against pain.

Functional MRI studies offer another layer of insight by showing decreased activity in the default mode network (DMN) during mindfulness meditation. The DMN, often active during mind-wandering and self-referential thinking, can contribute to heightened emotional responses to pain. When its activity decreases, individuals report less emotional distress related to pain episodes, allowing them to experience discomfort without the added layer of anxiety or rumination that can exacerbate their condition (Zeidan et al., 2019).

The reduction in DMN activity exemplifies how mindfulness can lower emotional reactivity to pain, providing a more stable mental state. This stability helps in reframing pain not as an overwhelming threat but as a manageable experience. By decreasing the emotional load carried with pain, mindfulness practitioners often find themselves less consumed by the fear or depression that may accompany chronic conditions.

As mindfulness continues to become a popular component of pain management strategies, it's important for those suffering from chronic pain to understand how these practices can biologically and psychologically uplift them. Mindful attention to the present moment offers a reprieve from the cycle of negativity that chronic pain can enforce, creating space for healing and adaptation.

In essence, the practice of mindfulness in managing pain draws from its ability to foster meaningful changes in brain function. Whether through enhanced connectivity within pain-regulating areas, modulation of neurotransmitter levels, or reduced activity in neural networks associated with emotional distress, mindfulness offers a multi-faceted approach to pain management. By embracing these practices, individuals may discover newfound pathways to cope with and ultimately transcend their pain.

Research Studies on Pain Reduction

The exploration of mindfulness as a tool for managing chronic pain has gained significant traction within the scientific community. Recent meta-analyses shed light on its moderate effectiveness in comparison to other interventions. These studies underscore the potential benefits of integrating mindfulness into treatment plans, as they reveal consistent patterns of pain reduction among participants who engage in such practices.

In particular, mindfulness-based interventions (MBIs) have been shown to yield statistically significant results in randomized controlled trials (RCTs). Participants often report noticeable reductions in pain intensity after practicing mindfulness techniques, with these effects tending to persist long after the conclusion of the interventions. This suggests that mindfulness not only mitigates immediate pain but also equips individuals with skills to manage their pain in the long term. Such findings illustrate how mindfulness can serve as a sustainable adjunct to traditional pain management approaches.

Longitudinal studies provide additional insights into the enduring benefits of mindfulness for individuals experiencing chronic pain. These studies have observed sustained pain relief and psychological improvements months after completing mindfulness training programs. By helping reduce the recurrence of pain flares, mindfulness training supports the idea that regular practice can instill lasting resilience and adaptability in coping with chronic conditions. Notably, this extended benefit positions mindfulness as a valuable tool not just for immediate relief, but for long-term well-being and quality of life enhancement.

Specific conditions, such as fibromyalgia and chronic back pain, are particularly responsive to mindfulness practices. Research indicates that mindfulness not only alleviates physical symptoms but also addresses the psychological components that exacerbate these conditions. For instance, mindfulness helps diminish anxiety-related pain amplification—a common issue among those with fibromyalgia. By fostering a sense of calm and detachment from anxious thoughts, mindfulness reduces the overall burden of pain for sufferers.

To understand why mindfulness is effective, it's crucial to consider its holistic impact on both mind and body. Mindfulness encourages individuals to focus on the present moment, recognizing and accepting their pain without judgment or aversion. This shift in perspective facilitates a decrease in stress, which often contributes to heightened pain perception. Moreover, by emphasizing non-reactivity and awareness, mindfulness promotes psychological flexibility—a key factor in managing chronic pain's unpredictability.

These scientific insights reveal a clear pattern: mindfulness emerges as a promising avenue for reducing chronic pain across diverse contexts and populations. It empowers individuals with tools that extend beyond temporary relief, fostering an enduring transformation in how they experience and handle pain. As evidence accumulates, it strengthens the case for integrating mindfulness into comprehensive pain management strategies, offering new hope for those seeking alternatives to conventional treatments.

Overall, the growing body of research highlights that mindfulness offers more than mere symptom relief; it represents a paradigm shift in understanding and addressing chronic pain. As the field continues to evolve, there is potential for mindfulness to become a cornerstone in pain management, empowering individuals to reclaim their quality of life through sustained psychological and physical well-being.

Mindfulness and Brain Function

Mindfulness practices have been increasingly recognized for their ability to reshape cognitive functions, particularly in the context of pain perception and stress management. At the core of this transformation is the concept of cognitive flexibility, which refers to the ability to adapt one's thinking and behavior in response to changing circumstances. Mindfulness enhances this cognitive agility by fostering an awareness that allows individuals to observe their thoughts nonjudgmentally. When applied to pain management, this increased flexibility enables individuals to manage negative thoughts surrounding pain more effectively, promoting adaptive coping strategies that can mitigate the emotional distress often accompanying chronic pain.

A study by Gary Charness et al. (2024) highlights how mindfulness training contributes to cognitive flexibility, showing significant improvements in participants' ability to navigate stress and cognitive demands effectively. This cognitive enhancement allows those with chronic pain to reassess their relationship with pain, moving from a reactive to a proactive approach. By doing so, individuals can break free from the cycle of rumination and negative thought patterns that exacerbate pain, instead cultivating resilience and acceptance.

Moreover, mindfulness plays a pivotal role in improving focus and attention, key components in managing pain and enhancing overall well-being. By practicing mindfulness, individuals learn to direct their attention deliberately, reducing the automatic nature of attentional drift that often accompanies chronic pain conditions. This intentional focusing ability helps distract from pain sensations, allowing individuals to redirect their energy toward positive activities and thoughts that foster resilience. The work of Lazar et al. (2005) supports this by showing how mindfulness leads to increased thickness in brain regions implicated in attention and sensory processing, such as the prefrontal cortex and right anterior insula. These neural changes underline how mindfulness practice not only alters cognitive processes but also leads to structural modifications in the brain, aiding in effective pain distraction.

Another significant benefit of mindfulness is its impact on working memory performance, which is crucial for learning new coping strategies for pain management. Working memory allows individuals to hold information temporarily while integrating it with long-term knowledge, a process essential for developing effective pain management techniques. Through mindfulness, individuals enhance their working memory capacity, leading to improved comprehension and application of new strategies that can alleviate pain. This enhancement is further supported by evidence suggesting that mindfulness training increases gray matter concentration in brain areas active during meditation (Hölzel et al., 2008), indicating neuroplastic changes that bolster working memory function.

In addition, mindfulness has a profound effect on decision-making capabilities, which play a critical role in pain management. Mindfulness encourages a careful weighing of options, allowing individuals to approach pain-related decisions with greater clarity and less emotional interference. By cultivating a nonreactive stance to thoughts and emotions, mindfulness helps individuals assess their situations objectively, facilitating more considered and effective decision-making regarding pain interventions and lifestyle adjustments. This aligns with findings by Keng et al. (2011), who note how mindfulness fosters nonjudgmental awareness, promoting psychological health and resilience.

The interplay between mindfulness and cognitive functions underscores a transformative potential that extends beyond mere symptom relief. By reshaping cognitive processes such as flexibility, focus, working memory, and decision-making, mindfulness offers a comprehensive framework for addressing the multifaceted challenges of chronic pain. As individuals harness these enhanced cognitive abilities, they gain access to a toolset that empowers them to engage with their condition proactively, ultimately improving their quality of life. This cognitive shift not only aids in managing the immediate effects of pain but also equips individuals with long-term strategies that contribute to sustained well-being and reduced dependence on medical interventions.

Impact on Stress and Anxiety

In the realm of pain management, mindfulness emerges as a beacon of hope, offering scientifically backed strategies for alleviating chronic discomfort. This chapter subpoints focus on the intricate relationship between mindfulness and its capacity to reduce stress and anxiety—factors that directly influence our perception of pain.

A fundamental understanding begins with recognizing how stress exacerbates physical discomfort. When we're stressed, our body's natural response is to tighten, increasing muscle tension and, consequently, our sensitivity to pain. The body's stress response, often referred to as "fight or flight," triggers a cascade of physiological reactions designed to protect us in emergencies. However, chronic activation of this response can lead to persistent muscle tension, which amplifies pain sensations, leading to a vicious cycle of discomfort (Bentley et al., 2023).

Mindfulness techniques offer a powerful counterbalance by reducing these physiological markers of stress. Through practices like mindful breathing and meditation, individuals can learn to calm their body's nervous system, thereby reducing muscle tension. Regular mindfulness practice has been shown to be effective not only in reducing physiological stress markers but also in minimizing the overall impact stress has on the body (Toussaint et al., 2021).

Psychologically, mindfulness serves as an anchor amid turbulent thoughts. Chronic pain often brings an unwelcome companion: anxiety. Anxious thoughts about the future or regrets about the past can exacerbate one's experience of pain, making it feel more intense and less manageable. Mindfulness empowers individuals to detach from these anxious narratives, fostering a sense of calm and presence. Practitioners learn to observe their thoughts without judgment, creating space between stimulus and response. This detachment allows them to experience pain without the additional layer of anxiety-driven interpretation, effectively diminishing the psychological distress associated with pain.

Central to mindfulness's effectiveness in stress relief are strategies like voluntary regulated breathing practices. These include diaphragmatic breathing, paced slow breathing, and alternate-nostril breathing, each offering unique benefits. Such techniques can significantly lower the body's reactivity to stress, activating the parasympathetic nervous system, known for promoting relaxation (Bentley et al., 2023). Individuals can integrate these practices into daily routines, using them as immediate tools to regain composure during heightened moments of stress.

As stress levels decrease through mindful intervention, there is a notable shift in how pain is perceived and managed. Reduced stress not only correlates with lower reported pain ratings but also translates to decreased reliance on pain medication, a significant benefit for those seeking alternative pain management methods. By cultivating mindfulness, individuals empower themselves to proactively manage stress, potentially leading to fewer medical interventions and improving their overall quality of life (Toussaint et al., 2021).

This holistic approach to pain management underscores mindfulness's capacity to address both the mind and the body's needs. Mindfulness provides real-world applications, extending beyond theoretical benefits into practical strategies that empower individuals to take control of their well-being. In doing so, practitioners cultivate resilience, harnessing the power of the present moment to break free from the shackles of chronic pain. This empowering journey towards self-awareness and acceptance illustrates mindfulness's pivotal role in redefining one's relationship with pain.

Evidence-Based Benefits

Mindfulness is a practice rooted in ancient traditions, yet its relevance and applicability to modern health challenges, particularly chronic pain management, have become increasingly supported by scientific studies. The wisdom of mindfulness fosters acceptance rather than avoidance, empowering individuals to approach pain with a sense of openness and resilience. This shift is crucial as it counters the natural human tendency to resist or deny discomfort, which often exacerbates suffering.

Acceptance through mindfulness involves recognizing pain as a part of one's experience without judgment. By cultivating an awareness that includes pain but does not define oneself by it, sufferers can alter their perceptions, reducing the impact of the pain on their daily lives. Studies highlight this ability to reshape responses to pain, offering a pathway to recovery and resilience (Zeidan & Vago, 2016).

Beyond individual psychological benefits, regular mindfulness practice contributes significantly to emotional well-being and an improved quality of life. Chronic pain frequently comes hand-in-hand with feelings of despair, anxiety, and social withdrawal. Yet, engaging consistently in mindfulness practices helps manage these emotions, fostering a more balanced mental state. Participants in mindfulness programs often report enhancements in their interpersonal relationships, as they learn not only to be more present within themselves but also to extend this presence to others around them. They begin to interact with loved ones more patiently and attentively, building stronger, empathetic connections (Sodeman, 2020).

The integration of mindfulness-based interventions into clinical settings marks a significant advancement in the holistic treatment of chronic pain. These interventions complement traditional medical treatments, forming a comprehensive plan that addresses both the physical and mental aspects of pain. Clinics incorporating mindfulness into their therapy regimens find an amplified treatment effectiveness as patients gain tools for self-regulation and enjoy reduced stress levels. Mindful breathing techniques, body scans, and meditation practices are just a few of the methods used to help patients regain control and reduce dependency on medications (Zeidan & Vago, 2016).

Another noteworthy benefit of mindfulness lies in its social dimension. Group sessions provide opportunities for community building among individuals who otherwise might feel isolated due to their conditions. These sessions create supportive environments where participants can share experiences and strategies, fostering a sense of belonging. As they meditate together and discuss their challenges and victories, participants build networks that help them to combat isolation — a common consequence of chronic pain. The camaraderie and mutual support found in these groups not only bolster individual spirits but also contribute to overall mental health improvement, showing that shared mindfulness experiences can be powerful antidotes to loneliness (Sodeman, 2020).

In summary, mindfulness presents numerous documented benefits for managing chronic pain effectively. It enables acceptance over avoidance, teaches us how to live more fully in each moment despite discomfort, and strengthens emotional resilience. At the same time, it improves personal relationships and integrates seamlessly into broader treatment plans, demonstrating remarkable results when used alongside other therapeutic modalities. Moreover, the community aspect of mindfulness offers considerable social benefits, reducing the isolation that often accompanies chronic pain and helping sufferers reclaim a sense of community and purpose in their lives.

Summary and Reflections

The chapter has explored the fascinating intersection of mindfulness and pain management, shedding light on how these practices can lead to profound changes in both mind and body. By engaging specific brain regions and enhancing connectivity across areas involved in pain regulation, mindfulness reshapes our experience of pain from a place of despair to one of empowerment. It encourages a focus on the present, therefore reducing stress and emotional distress that often accompany chronic pain. Mindfulness doesn't just aim for temporary relief; instead, it equips individuals with tools for long-lasting transformation, promoting resilience and emotional well-being even as they navigate the complexities of chronic conditions.

As we've seen, the research supporting mindfulness is encouraging and underscores its potential as a vital component of comprehensive pain management strategies. Regular practice can decrease reliance on medications and foster psychological flexibility, helping individuals adapt to the unpredictability of their condition. Through building awareness and acceptance, mindfulness opens pathways to healing and adaptation, enhancing quality of life and providing hope for those seeking to reclaim their lives from chronic pain's grasp. This journey toward mindfulness offers not just a method but a way of living that transforms struggles into opportunities for growth and renewal.

Reference List

Bentley, T. G. K., D'Andrea-Penna, G., Rakic, M., Arce, N., LaFaille, M., Berman, R., Cooley, K., & Sprimont, P. (2023, November 21). *Breathing Practices for Stress and Anxiety Reduction: Conceptual Framework of Implementation Guidelines Based on a Systematic Review of the Published Literature.* Brain Sciences. https://doi.org/10.3390/brainsci13121612

Charness, G., Le Bihan, Y., & Villeval, M. C. (2024, January 1). *Mindfulness training, cognitive performance and stress reduction.* Journal of Economic Behavior & Organization. https://doi.org/10.1016/j.jebo.2023.10.027

Calderone, A., Latella, D., Impellizzeri, F., Pasquale, P. de, Famà, F., Quartarone, A., & Calabrò, R. S. (2024, November 15). *Neurobiological Changes Induced by Mindfulness and Meditation: A Systematic Review.* Biomedicines; Multidisciplinary Digital Publishing Institute. https://doi.org/10.3390/biomedicines12112613

Keng, S. L., Smoski, M. J., & Robins, C. J. (2011). *Effects of Mindfulness on Psychological health: a Review of Empirical Studies.* Clinical Psychology Review. https://doi.org/10.1016/j.cpr.2011.04.006

Sodeman, L. (2020, September 25). *Use mindfulness to cope with chronic pain.* Www.mayoclinichealthsystem.org. https://www.mayoclinichealthsystem.org/hometown-health/speaking-of-health/use-mindfulness-to-cope-with-chronic-pain

Toussaint, L., Nguyen, Q. A., Roettger, C., Dixon, K., Offenbächer, M., Kohls, N., Hirsch, J., & Sirois, F. (2021). *Effectiveness of Progressive Muscle Relaxation, Deep Breathing, and Guided Imagery in Promoting Psychological and Physiological States of Relaxation* (R. Taylor-Piliae, Ed.). Evidence-Based Complementary and Alternative Medicine. https://doi.org/10.1155/2021/5924040

Veehof, M. M., Trompetter, H. R., Bohlmeijer, E. T., & Schreurs, K. M. G. (2016, January 2). *Acceptance- and mindfulness-based interventions for the treatment of chronic pain: a meta-analytic review.* Cognitive Behaviour Therapy. https://doi.org/10.1080/16506073.2015.1098724

Zeidan, F., & Vago, D. R. (2016, June). *Mindfulness meditation-based pain relief: a mechanistic account.* Annals of the New York Academy of Sciences. https://doi.org/10.1111/nyas.13153

Zhang, D., Lee, E. K. P., Mak, E. C. W., Ho, C. Y., & Wong, S. Y. S. (2021). *Mindfulness-based interventions: An overall review.* British Medical Bulletin. https://doi.org/10.1093/bmb/ldab005

Zeidan, F., Baumgartner, J. N., & Coghill, R. C. (2019). *The neural mechanisms of mindfulness-based pain relief.* PAIN Reports. https://doi.org/10.1097/pr9.0000000000000759

CHAPTER 3

Mindfulness Techniques for Pain Reduction

Reducing pain through mindfulness techniques can offer a transformative experience for those living with chronic discomfort. By focusing on the present moment and cultivating awareness of one's breath, body, and mind, mindfulness becomes a practical tool in managing pain more effectively. It encourages sufferers to create a buffer between themselves and their pain, promoting a calm and focused state of being that can diminish distress. The essence of mindfulness lies not in eradicating pain but redefining how one interacts with it, thus altering its impact on daily life.

In this chapter, readers will discover various mindfulness exercises specifically designed for pain management. Breathing techniques such as Deep Belly Breathing and 4-7-8 Breathing will be explored, offering methods to harness the power of breath in calming the body and mind. Additionally, the chapter delves into Body Scan Meditation, providing insights on identifying tension without judgment, which can lead to relief over time. Mindful movement practices like Gentle Yoga and Tai Chi are also discussed, highlighting their potential to enhance flexibility and reduce anxiety. Lastly, Guided Imagery will reveal how visualization of soothing scenes can redirect focus from pain, fostering a sense of control and tranquility. Through these exercises, individuals will learn how to integrate mindfulness into everyday activities, ultimately improving their quality of life despite the ongoing challenges of chronic pain.

Breathing Techniques

In the realm of pain management, breathing techniques provide a gateway to relief by fostering relaxation and focus. For individuals grappling with chronic pain, these practices offer both a physical and mental shift that can significantly ease discomfort.

To begin with, Deep Belly Breathing is a simple yet powerful technique that activates your body's natural relaxation response. Unlike shallow chest breathing, which often occurs during stress, this method involves taking slow, deep breaths. As you inhale deeply through your nose, imagine filling not just your lungs but your entire belly with air. This action encourages the diaphragm to move down, expanding the belly outward. A noticeable benefit here is the reduction of tension. By engaging in Deep Belly Breathing regularly, you can train your body to instinctively resort to this calming practice, particularly in moments of heightened pain or anxiety (Ankrom, 2024).

Another technique, 4-7-8 Breathing, serves as a rhythmic pattern that grounds the mind and provides emotional stability. It's especially helpful when you're lying awake at night, with worries magnifying your perception of pain. The process entails inhaling through your nose for four seconds, holding your breath for seven, and then exhaling fully through your mouth for eight seconds. The rhythmic nature distracts from pain sensations, shifting focus to the task of breathing itself. Over time, you'll find a decrease in overall anxiety levels, offering a much-needed reprieve for a racing mind (Gotter, 2018).

For those seeking mental clarity alongside pain relief, Alternate Nostril Breathing stands out. This ancient yogic practice balances the energies within your body and soothes the mind, reducing feelings of anxiety. To perform it, sit comfortably and use your right thumb to close off your right nostril, inhaling through the left. Then, close the left nostril with your ring finger and exhale through the right. Continue alternating in this manner. Beyond its calming effects, practitioners often report an enhanced sense of awareness and improved mental clarity, crucial for anyone navigating the complexities of chronic pain (Telles et al., 2017).

Integrating mindfulness into everyday activities is possible through Mindful Breathing During Activities. Whether you're washing dishes, taking a walk, or simply sitting in stillness, maintaining awareness of your breath fosters a connection between mind and body. This connection reduces stress and enhances your ability to manage pain. By focusing on each inhalation and exhalation, you remain rooted in the present moment, preventing your mind from wandering to past or future stressors. The beauty of this practice lies in its versatility—it can be seamlessly incorporated into any part of your day, making mindfulness an accessible tool for pain management.

Body Scan Meditation

In the realm of managing chronic pain, one valuable tool that stands out is body scan meditation. This practice teaches individuals to develop a non-judgmental awareness of their physical sensations, aiding in identifying areas of habitual tension that may contribute to discomfort. Through a gentle exploration of bodily sensations, participants are encouraged to become more present and mindful, recognizing pain without allowing it to overwhelm them.

At its core, the body scan technique is a simple yet profound exercise in paying attention to what is happening within your own body. It involves deliberately guiding your focus through different parts of the body, from head to toe, taking note of any sensation—be it tension, warmth, tightness, or even numbness—without judgment. The key here is not to label these sensations as good or bad, but to cultivate an acute awareness of them. Such awareness can often reveal underlying patterns of tension that might be intensified by stress or emotional turmoil, offering insights into how these elements interrelate with physical pain. By honing this skill, individuals can begin to address these tensions, possibly alleviating pain over time.

Guided Body Scan practices go further by providing structure and security during exploration. Novices might initially find the idea of tuning into uncomfortable sensations daunting. Guided meditations, often facilitated by experienced practitioners or recorded audio sessions, provide a sense of support, making the process more approachable. These guides lead the practitioner step-by-step, encouraging them to breathe deeply as they turn their attention inward, gently prompting them to notice and sit with each physical sensation, whether pleasant or not.

The true benefit of a guided body scan is the connection it fosters between mindfulness and pain management. As individuals learn to observe their pain rather than react to it, they can create a space where discomfort does not entirely dominate their experience. Instead, they perceive it as part of their body's communication system. With continued practice, this approach can reduce the distress associated with chronic pain by changing how one relates to the sensation itself. Mindfulness undermines the automatic reaction to push away or resist pain, fostering instead a more balanced and less fraught relationship with one's own body.

Integrating these short body scans into daily routines can also serve as effective stress relievers, enhancing emotional regulation. For instance, taking a few minutes each day to perform a quick body scan can interrupt the cycle of stress, allowing for a moment of introspection and calm. This kind of daily practice doesn't need to be lengthy; even a five-minute scan can provide significant benefits. By routinely engaging with the body in this way, individuals can better understand their emotional responses and reduce the impact of stressors that exacerbate pain. Regular body scans help fortify resilience against external pressures by promoting a mindful pause, a crucial tool for anyone grappling with ongoing physical discomfort.

Furthermore, the practice of self-compassion is inherently tied to body scans, nurturing an acceptance of oneself and transforming perceptions of pain. By acknowledging sensations without judgment, individuals start to break free from negative narratives about their bodies. This non-critical self-awareness nurtures a gentler internal dialogue, countering harsh self-judgments that often accompany chronic pain conditions. Through compassionate attention, the mind can slowly shift from being at odds with the body to becoming its ally. Over time, this shift facilitates a new perspective on pain—one that acknowledges discomfort as a transient experience rather than an inherent flaw.

Body scan meditation does more than just manage pain; it encourages a holistic approach to understanding and interacting with one's body and emotions. Practically speaking, integrating this mindfulness technique regularly fosters a deeper self-awareness and empowers individuals to respond to their needs with kindness and clarity (Raypole, 2020). For those dealing with chronic pain, this type of mindful interaction can significantly improve quality of life by building a foundation of trust and understanding with one's own body. In mastering the art of listening attentively to the body's cues, people can navigate their pain experiences with greater equanimity, reducing the overall psychological burden that often accompanies chronic conditions (Scott, 2024).

Mindful Movement Practices

In the realm of pain management, mindful movement exercises offer a promising pathway not only for reducing discomfort but also for enhancing mobility and overall quality of life. For individuals suffering from chronic pain, integrating these practices into daily routines can foster a deeper connection with their bodies, allowing for a more effective self-management strategy.

Gentle Yoga stands as one of the most accessible and beneficial mindful movement practices. This ancient discipline emphasizes the synchronization of breath with movement and encourages mindfulness by requiring practitioners to focus on each pose. Poses in gentle yoga are designed to improve flexibility and relieve muscle tension, two factors that can exacerbate chronic pain. By concentrating on maintaining proper posture and taking deep, deliberate breaths, individuals cultivate an awareness of their physical state, which helps them adjust and adapt movements to their comfort levels. It is essential during yoga sessions to listen closely to your body; if any pose leads to discomfort, modifications should be made or the pose avoided entirely. Practicing gentle yoga regularly can increase one's flexibility, balance, and overall body awareness—key aspects of managing chronic pain effectively (jason, 2024).

Meanwhile, Tai Chi offers a unique blend of graceful, flowing movements combined with meditation and deep breathing. Often referred to as "meditation in motion," this practice originates from ancient Chinese martial arts and serves as a potent tool for promoting balance and mindfulness. Its low-impact nature makes it highly suitable for all ages, including those dealing with chronic pain. The slow, deliberate movements help enhance coordination, reduce anxiety, and create a sense of inner peace. As you practice Tai Chi, focusing on the precise execution of movements and controlled breathing can lead to improved posture, increased circulation, and better stress management (*10 Types of Moving Meditations—Benefits of Mindful Movement | the Buddhist Center*, n.d.). These improvements contribute significantly to reducing the perception of pain and improving mobility.

Walking Meditation provides yet another approach to incorporating mindfulness into everyday activities. Unlike traditional walking, this practice involves moving at a slower pace and paying close attention to each step and the sensations within your body. It cultivates awareness of the present moment and creates a grounding effect, which can be particularly helpful for pain sufferers looking to connect more intimately with their bodies. It's less about reaching a destination and more about experiencing the journey with mindfulness. Walking meditation can alleviate depression and improve functional fitness while offering the dual benefits of better digestion and enhanced sleep quality (jason, 2024). Focusing on each step allows for a mental break from the cycle of pain thoughts, reinforcing the mind-body connection.

Finally, Integrating Movement into Daily Life is crucial for developing sustainable mindful habits that aid in managing chronic pain. Encouraging small, regular bursts of activity throughout the day can be transformative. For instance, simple stretches or gentle exercises upon waking can set a positive tone for the rest of the day. Being mindful during routine tasks such as standing up from a chair, lifting objects, or even washing dishes transforms these into opportunities for mini mindfulness exercises. This approach not only encourages active engagement in daily life but also underscores the idea that movement doesn't have to happen in a structured session to be beneficial. Consistently paying attention to how your body feels and moves supports an ongoing dialogue between mind and body, aiding in the alleviation of pain.

Guided Imagery for Relaxation

Guided imagery is a powerful technique that employs the mind's capacity to form vivid, soothing images, helping alleviate pain and cultivate a sense of calmness. This process involves visualizing positive scenes or experiences, which can effectively redirect focus from discomfort. When engaging in guided imagery, individuals are encouraged to conjure images that evoke comfort, such as lying on a warm beach or walking through a quiet forest, allowing them to shift their attention away from pain and towards these tranquil scenarios. This practice not only diminishes the perception of pain but also instills a feeling of control over one's pain experiences.

Creating personal scripts is an essential aspect of guided imagery, enabling individuals to tailor the visualization process for enhanced pain management. By crafting personalized narratives that incorporate specific imagery and sensory details, individuals gain autonomy over how they perceive and manage their pain. For instance, someone with chronic back pain might visualize waves gently massaging their spine, dispersing tension with each ebb and flow. These personal scripts act as mental blueprints, offering a unique and customizable approach to pain relief.

An integral component of guided imagery is utilizing nature scenarios, which leverages nature's inherent calming properties to induce relaxation and mitigate pain. Nature has long been recognized for its therapeutic effects, and incorporating it into guided imagery can amplify these benefits. Imagining oneself amidst a lush forest, with sunlight filtering through the leaves and birds chirping around, can transport the mind to a state of peace. Breathing in the imagined fresh air and feeling the gentle breeze can significantly reduce stress levels, promoting tranquility and reducing pain perceptions.

Integrating guided imagery into daily routine is crucial for maximizing its benefits and fortifying emotional resilience. Regular practice strengthens the mind-body connection, making it easier to access these visualizations during times of acute distress. Establishing a routine, such as setting aside time each morning or before bed, allows individuals to consistently engage in this therapeutic exercise. Over time, this regular engagement can lead to profound relaxation benefits, enhancing emotional stability and overall well-being. It also fosters a proactive approach to pain management, empowering individuals to utilize guided imagery as a dependable tool for alleviating discomfort and enhancing quality of life.

Developing Awareness of Pain

Understanding and managing chronic pain through mindfulness invites a transformative approach, focusing on the profound relationship between mind and body. At the heart of this lies the concept of mindfulness and its impact on pain perception, which enables individuals to distinguish between the physical sensation of pain and their emotional response to it. This differentiation can significantly reduce the psychological burden often associated with chronic pain.

The ancient practice of mindfulness meditation has long been reputed for modifying how pain is perceived. By teaching individuals to fully experience the sensory component of pain without evaluating or reacting emotionally, mindfulness reduces the layers of suffering added by our minds (Zeidan & Vago, 2016). This reduction in emotional reactivity can lead to a more manageable pain experience, as we begin to understand that the sensation of pain itself may not be as distressing without the accompanying emotional turmoil.

Mindfulness practices such as open-monitoring meditation encourage an attentive awareness of thoughts and emotions as they arise, without judgment. This method allows practitioners to observe their pain sensations straightforwardly, acknowledging them without allowing subsequent emotional reactions to amplify their intensity (Lu et al., 2023). As individuals become more adept at this practice, they report feeling less bothered by their pain, finding themselves able to engage more fully in life despite their discomfort.

Journaling pain experiences offers another layer of understanding, serving as a tool to clarify thought patterns related to pain and identify potential triggers. The process of recording these experiences doesn't just provide clarity but also aids in self-advocacy when seeking medical treatments. By keeping track of fluctuations in pain and associated triggers, individuals can present a comprehensive picture to healthcare providers, facilitating accurate diagnosis and treatment plans tailored to their needs. Encouraging readers to establish a routine of noting down their daily pain experiences, alongside emotional states and external factors, can unveil hidden patterns and contribute to more informed management strategies.

Regular check-ins with pain assist individuals in developing compassionate responses over reactive ones. Instead of immediately resorting to habitual reactions like frustration or avoidance, these check-ins promote a kinder dialogue with one's own body. Such mindful inquiry encourages patience and empathy towards oneself, fostering a deeper understanding of body signals. This practice involves setting aside time each day to quietly observe any discomfort, examining its qualities without judgement. By doing so, people cultivate an attitude of acceptance, allowing them to respond to their pain constructively and adaptively.

Additionally, distinguishing between types of pain plays a crucial role in targeted management. Chronic pain, which persists over extended periods, demands different strategies compared to temporary pain. Recognizing these distinctions helps in forming appropriate responses and treatment plans. Mindfulness can further these efforts by drawing attention to the emotional connections tied to various types of pain, highlighting how mental and emotional states may exacerbate or alleviate physical sensations.

One practical aspect of differentiating pain types is considering their origins. For example, muscle strain might present differently from nerve-related pain, and both require distinct approaches for relief. Understanding emotional undercurrents is equally important—stress and anxiety can intensify perceived pain levels, while relaxation and positive thinking may serve as natural analgesics.

By cultivating awareness through mindfulness and journaling, individuals can familiarize themselves with these nuances, leading to personalized interventions that align with their specific circumstances. Despite the complexity of chronic pain, this approach empowers individuals to take control of their management strategies, enhancing autonomy and improving quality of life.

Final Thoughts

This chapter has gently taken you through the world of practical mindfulness exercises crafted specifically for pain management. By exploring breathing techniques, such as Deep Belly Breathing and 4-7-8 Breathing, you discovered methods to foster relaxation and focus, helping to ease the grip of chronic pain. The journey continued with body scan meditation, nurturing a non-judgmental awareness of your physical sensations. This mindful practice revealed how recognizing pain without overwhelming emotion can gradually reduce the impact of discomfort. Additionally, mindful movement practices like gentle yoga and Tai Chi offered ways to harmonize breath and movement, enhancing mobility and reducing anxiety.

Guided imagery provided another path, where visualizing soothing scenes took precedence over pain, crafting a mental sanctuary. Meanwhile, developing an acute awareness of pain through open-monitoring meditation helped distinguish between physical sensations and emotional reactions. Each section emphasized empowering strategies to handle daily challenges, inviting you to deepen your connection with yourself. As you integrate these practices into your life, remember that they are not just tools but companions on your journey to reclaim a sense of control and improve your quality of life. Embrace this newfound understanding and move forward with compassion and patience toward peace and healing.

Reference List

10 Types of Moving Meditations—Benefits of Mindful Movement | The Buddhist Center. (n.d.). Tnlsf.org. https://tnlsf.org/10-types-of-moving-meditations-benefits-of-mindful-movement/

Ankrom, S. (2024, February 16). *Need a Breather? Try These 9 Breathing Exercises to Relieve Anxiety*. Verywell Mind. https://www.verywellmind.com/abdominal-breathing-2584115

Benefits of Guided Imagery for Pain Management | Beaumont | Beaumont Health. (n.d.). Www.beaumont.org. https://www.beaumont.org/services/pain-management-services/benefits-of-guided-imagery-for-pain-management

Gotter, A. (2018, April 20). *What Is the 4-7-8 Breathing Technique?* Healthline; Healthline Media. https://www.healthline.com/health/4-7-8-breathing

Lu, C., Moliadze, V., & Nees, F. (2023, November 9). *Dynamic processes of mindfulness-based alterations in pain perception*. Frontiers in Neuroscience; Frontiers Media. https://doi.org/10.3389/fnins.2023.1253559

Raypole, C. (2020, March 26). *Body Scan Meditation: Benefits and How to Do It*. Healthline. https://www.healthline.com/health/body-scan-meditation

Scott, E. (2024, February 12). *What is body scan meditation?* Verywell Mind. https://www.verywellmind.com/body-scan-meditation-why-and-how-3144782

Visualization & Guided Imagery for Pain Relief (The Complete Guide) - Pathways. (2020, May 30). Www.pathways.health. https://www.pathways.health/blog/visualization-guided-imagery-for-pain-relief/

Zeidan, F., & Vago, D. R. (2016, June). *Mindfulness meditation-based pain relief: a mechanistic account*. Annals of the New York Academy of Sciences. https://doi.org/10.1111/nyas.13153

jason. (2024, October 23). *5 Mindful Movement Practices for Optimal Health and Well-Being - Health & Wellness Canada*. Health & Wellness Canada. https://www.healthcouncilcanada.ca/5-mindful-movement-practices-for-optimal-health-and-well-being/

CHAPTER 4

Developing a Daily
Mindfulness Practice

Developing a daily mindfulness practice is about creating moments where the mind can pause amidst the chaos of daily life. For individuals who live with chronic pain, these moments are more than just brief respites; they are opportunities to foster a sense of inner peace and presence amidst their struggles. Mindfulness allows us to focus on the now, offering a gentle pathway toward understanding and coping with discomfort. It invites curiosity instead of judgment and opens the door to embracing each moment with compassion. This chapter uncovers how tapping into this silent awareness through everyday activities can transform routines into chances for renewal and growth.

As routines become second nature, this chapter will explore essential steps that gently guide you through integrating mindfulness into daily life. From setting clear intentions to creating spaces that nurture tranquility, you will learn techniques that support a sustainable practice. Maintaining balance requires adaptability, and the guidance offered here will show how to manifest mindfulness even in simple tasks. Each step brings new ways to engage with life's rhythm, helping to align practices with personal needs and enhance emotional well-being. Discover how mindful transitions, consistent habits, and personalized rituals can turn ordinary days into extraordinary journeys, promoting healing at every turn.

Setting Intentions

Setting intentions within the practice of mindfulness serves as a foundation for cultivating a more focused and purposeful life, especially for individuals living with chronic pain. Intentions act as guiding stars, offering both direction and motivation in the often challenging journey of managing pain. An intention is not about achieving specific outcomes but about fostering a mindful state and deeper engagement with one's own experience. As you set intentions, they become a source of empowerment, reinforcing personal agency and encouraging self-exploration regarding how you wish to live and interact with the world.

At the heart of setting intentions is the creation of a structure that aligns your daily actions with broader healing objectives. When intentions are clearly defined, they foster a sense of accountability, enabling you to align your efforts with your overarching goals for pain management and well-being. Such clarity ensures that every action taken is purposefully connected to a larger narrative, enhancing coherence and consistency in one's mindfulness practice. This sense of accountability encourages individuals to stay committed, even when faced with setbacks, by reminding them of their larger aspirations and the progress made toward them.

Personalizing intentions plays a critical role in strengthening engagement. Each individual's experience with chronic pain is unique, thus requiring tailored approaches to mindfulness. By customizing intentions, you ensure they resonate deeply with your personal journey and cater specifically to your needs and circumstances. For instance, you might set an intention centered around embracing moments of discomfort with compassion—recognizing that such experiences are part of your path to healing. This personalized approach anchors intentions in the reality of your situation, making them more relevant and impactful on your day-to-day practices.

Reflection is another essential aspect of maintaining effective and meaningful intentions. Regularly revisiting and contemplating your intentions allows you to assess their relevance and effectiveness. Over time, as circumstances and perspectives shift, reflecting on intentions helps them evolve, adapting to your current state of being and aspirations. This continuous cycle of review fosters both personal growth and a deeper understanding of oneself, as it encourages introspection and the willingness to adjust one's mindset and approach to better suit present realities.

Creating mindful affirmations also complements the process of setting intentions. By framing intentions positively, you nurture a constructive and hopeful mindset, which is crucial for those seeking to navigate the complexities of chronic pain. Affirmations like "I embrace each moment with acceptance" or "I am open to growth and healing" serve as constant reminders of your commitment to living mindfully and resiliently. These affirmations reinforce the emotional and mental fortitude required to engage with daily challenges while staying true to your path of healing.

Guidelines for crafting these affirmations include simplicity and positivity. Keeping affirmations straightforward prevents them from becoming overwhelming or diluted in meaning. Simplicity helps maintain focus and ensures that the affirmation remains a strong anchor in moments of need. Additionally, focusing on positive language steers attention away from limitations and towards possibilities, fostering an empowering outlook that supports healing and well-being.

Examples of mindful intentions can offer inspiration and assist in the personalization process. Consider intentions like "I express gratitude for my body's resilience" or "I cultivate patience and kindness towards myself." These examples show how intentions can be linked to self-care practices and emotional resilience, emphasizing appreciation and self-compassion as key elements of managing chronic pain. Furthermore, they highlight the importance of recognizing and celebrating even small victories, as these contribute significantly to the overall journey of mindfulness.

Incorporating regular reflection on these intentions ensures they remain aligned with your evolving needs and goals. Set aside time to revisit your intentions, examining whether they continue to serve your current objectives. Ask yourself if they still resonate and reflect on any necessary adjustments. This practice not only maintains the relevance of your intentions but also supports ongoing personal development and growth.

Creating a Mindfulness Space

Creating a physical environment that supports mindfulness involves crafting an atmosphere that fosters tranquility, focus, and connection. A well-considered space can significantly enhance the efficacy of mindfulness practices by offering a sanctuary of calm in our bustling world.

Elements of a Mindfulness Space

To establish a conducive environment for mindfulness, key components should work together to create a calming atmosphere. This begins with minimizing distractions, which is crucial in helping you maintain focus during meditation or reflection. Choose colors, textures, and objects that evoke serenity and promote ease. Soft, natural hues often generate a soothing effect, reducing anxiety and leading the mind toward peace. (How, 2024)

Lighting also plays a significant role; avoid harsh overhead lights that may strain your eyes or disrupt your concentration. Instead, opt for soft illumination from lamps, dimmable lights, or candles that can cast a gentle glow over your space, setting a tranquil mood. Incorporating elements such as calming sounds—like gentle music or nature sounds—can further draw you into relaxation and help mask unwanted noise from the outside world. (Mate, 2024)

Personalizing the Space

Turning your mindfulness area into a personal retreat not only fosters comfort but deepens your connection to the practice. Personalization encourages ownership of the space, making it a more inviting refuge each time you return. Consider adorning your sanctuary with items that hold personal meaning—whether they are photographs, artwork, favorite books, or inspirational quotes. These elements reflect your individuality and serve as visual anchors, reminding you of your intentions and goals. (Mate, 2024)

Incorporating nature into your serene area can also bolster the feeling of tranquility and connection. Plants, stones, or other natural materials link you to the earth, providing grounding energy that aids in centering your thoughts. A small indoor plant like a peace lily or succulent not only livens up the environment but connects you subtly to nature's cycles, enhancing mindfulness naturally. The simplicity and balance provided by these natural elements emphasize the philosophy of mindfulness: living in harmony with oneself and one's surroundings. (How, 2024)

Location Considerations

Selecting the right location for your mindfulness space is essential in developing consistent practice habits. Ideally, find a spot that is quiet, away from high-traffic areas or sources of interruption. This ensures minimal disturbance, allowing your mind to settle and focus during sessions. Whether it's a corner in your living room or a dedicated room, the location should be easily accessible yet shielded enough to offer privacy and solitude.

When choosing your space, consider its versatility too. Think about how it can accommodate various mindful activities, from meditation to yoga or journaling, without needing constant adjustment. A flexible space adapts to different needs, fostering a habitual routine and encouraging frequent engagement with your mindfulness practices. (Mate, 2024)

Maintaining the Space

Regular maintenance of your mindfulness environment is crucial in keeping it inviting and signaling readiness for practice. Keeping the area tidy and free of clutter prevents visual distractions and promotes mental clarity. Establishing a simple routine to clean and organize the space ensures it remains a place you're eager to retreat to daily.

Occasional refreshment of the space can also rejuvenate your practice. Rotating decorative items, adding seasonal accents, or introducing new scents with candles or essential oils can revitalize the ambiance, aligning your environment with changing moods or preferences. It's essential to periodically assess whether each element genuinely enhances your mindfulness journey, ensuring the space continues to meet your evolving needs. (Mate, 2024)

Daily Mindful Routines

Integrating mindfulness into everyday activities allows individuals to cultivate sustained practice, a crucial component for those dealing with chronic pain. By finding presence in every task, we turn routine chores into opportunities for mindfulness exercises. Whether it's washing dishes or making the bed, each activity can become a chance to foster a deeper connection with the present moment. This approach not only helps manage pain but also enriches daily living.

Consider the simple act of washing dishes. Instead of viewing it as a mundane chore, consider it an exercise in mindfulness. Feel the warm water on your hands and focus on each dish's texture. This deliberate engagement transforms the task into a calming ritual, as explained by Thich Nhat Hanh in "The Miracle of Mindfulness" (Deschene, 2010). Embracing these daily rituals as opportunities for mindfulness allows moments that might otherwise feel tedious to become enriching parts of the day.

Creating consistent routines is another effective strategy for enhancing familiarity with mindfulness tools. Consistency fosters habit, embedding practices more deeply into daily life. Setting aside a few minutes each morning to engage in mindful breathing or savoring a hot drink without distractions can create a rhythm that permeates the day. Through this practice, mindfulness becomes second nature, steadily weaving its way throughout various aspects of life.

Mindful transitions provide yet another path toward integrating mindfulness into daily routines. These moments between tasks are often overlooked, yet they offer rich opportunities for reflection and emotional awareness. For instance, pausing for a breath between meetings or taking a moment to gather thoughts before starting a new activity can ease routine changes, prevent stress buildup, and enhance emotional clarity. Being conscious of these transitions helps maintain mindfulness throughout the day, minimizing the rush and chaos that may exacerbate pain and anxiety.

Scheduling specific time slots for mindfulness practice further aligns this practice with self-care commitments. By prioritizing dedicated time for mindfulness, much like setting an appointment for exercise or a doctor's visit, individuals affirm that caring for their mental well-being is essential. Establishing regular time slots for these practices strengthens commitment and ensures that mindfulness remains a central part of one's life rather than a sidelined intention.

Incorporating mindfulness into common tasks bridges the gap between a busy lifestyle and the need for mindful presence. Transforming routine activities like cooking or cleaning into moments of meditation offers a practical, inviting avenue for those seeking to improve quality of life while managing chronic pain. The gentle rhythm of slicing vegetables or sweeping the floor can become a dance of awareness, grounding one's mind in the current experience, much like how Ayesha Calligraphy describes the transformative potential of housework (Calligraphy, 2024).

Establishing consistent routines enhances the effectiveness of mindfulness tools. Repeating practices over time deepens familiarity and solidifies their place in daily life. Simple activities such as morning stretches or evening

67

reflections gradually build resilience and bring about noticeable improvements in emotional regulation and pain perception. These routines ground individuals in their commitment to mindfulness, offering a reliable structure amid the unpredictability of daily life.

Transition times pose unique opportunities for mindfulness. The brief pause between activities, when used mindfully, aids in emotional regulation and prepares the mind for the next task. These moments allow for a reset, providing space to check in with one's emotions and physical state. This heightened awareness contributes to smoother transitions, reducing the stress and discomfort associated with change, which is especially relevant in managing chronic pain.

Prioritizing mindfulness through scheduled practices serves as a powerful statement of commitment to self-care. Dedicating time in one's calendar for mindfulness-related activities leads to a consistent and focused practice. Intentional scheduling prevents mindfulness from being overshadowed by other responsibilities, reinforcing its importance in the overall strategy for pain management and mental wellness.

Recording Mindfulness Experiences

Embarking on a mindfulness journey often involves more than just the practice itself; it's also about documenting that journey to foster growth and reflection. One powerful tool in this process is a mindfulness journal, which serves multiple purposes in deepening one's awareness and providing motivational reminders of personal development.

A mindfulness journal acts as a mirror reflecting your inner world. Writing down thoughts and experiences can significantly increase self-awareness by capturing moments of clarity and obstacles faced in daily mindfulness practices (Egel, 2024). This tracking allows individuals to visually see their progress over time, which can be an inspiring motivator. For example, revisiting entries from weeks or months ago can illuminate the strides made in areas like emotional regulation or stress management, reinforcing the efficacy of your mindfulness practice.

Documenting emotional responses within a journal isn't merely about noting feelings but understanding their nuances and triggers. When you write about how certain mindfulness exercises affect you emotionally, it provides tangible evidence of what works best for you and underscores the practice's value. Such documentation highlights patterns that can lead to greater insights into behavioral changes and mental health improvements (allie, 2024). By making these observations visible, journals empower you to harness the most effective mindfulness tools for your unique needs.

Moreover, sharing insights from your mindfulness journal with others can create a sense of connection and community. The act of discussing your experiences not only offers support but also serves as a form of accountability. When others witness your journey—or take part in it—there's a mutual reinforcement that helps maintain dedication to the practice (Egel, 2024). Community engagement through shared journaling practices can reduce feelings of isolation and encourage collective growth, particularly beneficial for individuals managing chronic pain who value communal support.

Incorporating art and creativity into your journaling can further enrich personal understanding and engagement. Visual or creative outputs, such as drawings, poetry, or stream-of-consciousness entries, provide alternative ways to express thoughts and emotions that might be difficult to articulate with words alone. Artistic expression taps into different cognitive processes, fostering deeper emotional and spiritual connections (allie, 2024). When creativity is woven into mindfulness journaling, it transforms the experience into a dynamic narrative of personal exploration and discovery.

With various styles of mindfulness journals available, individuals can tailor their approaches to suit their preferences and goals. Some may prefer structured formats like gratitude or goal-setting journals, while others might lean toward freeform styles like sketchbooks or stream-of-consciousness writing. Finding the right format is crucial as it aligns your journaling practice with your personal objectives, enhancing the overall effectiveness of both mindfulness and journaling (Egel, 2024).

Adopting a regular journaling schedule, whether daily or weekly, establishes consistency—a cornerstone in any productive mindfulness practice. Yet, flexibility remains key, as personalization ensures that the journaling habit feels manageable and aligned with one's lifestyle. Regular journaling encourages introspection and continuous reflection, keeping the mind agile and mindful day by day.

As you engage with your mindfulness journal, consider setting clear intentions that guide your writing. Intentions might include cultivating self-awareness, reducing stress, or simply recording everyday reflections. Mindful journaling prompts can also serve as valuable tools, breaking writer's block and offering fresh perspectives. Questions like "What am I grateful for today?" or "What emotions did I experience during my meditation?" can help to structure entries, leading to deeper insights (allie, 2024).

This dedicated practice of documenting mindfulness fosters emotional intelligence and enhances personal growth, transforming one's approach to life's challenges. As each page fills, you build a reservoir of wisdom and experience that informs future decision-making and emotional resilience. Celebrating milestones noted in your journal can provide motivation and affirm the ongoing benefits of integrating mindfulness into daily life.

Overcoming Common Barriers

In the journey of developing a daily mindfulness practice, recognizing and overcoming common challenges is crucial. As individuals endeavor to integrate mindfulness into their lives, they often encounter barriers that can hinder progress. Understanding these obstacles—and how to address them—can significantly improve one's mindfulness journey.

Identifying personal obstacles is the first critical step in addressing these barriers effectively. Each person's experience is unique, and what might be perceived as a challenge to one person may not impact another similarly. For some, the obstacle may be a lack of time, where busy schedules seem to crowd out the possibility for mindful moments. Others might struggle with internal barriers such as negative self-talk or persistent rumination, which can distract from the focus needed in mindfulness practices. To navigate these challenges, individuals must engage in honest self-reflection to identify specific hurdles. By understanding one's personal obstacles, it becomes possible to devise strategies tailored to overcoming them, thus paving the way for a more consistent mindfulness practice.

One significant area that often requires attention is time management. Many people lead busy lives filled with work, family, and social commitments, leaving little room for new routines. However, by employing adaptable time management strategies, mindfulness can still find its place. This might involve setting aside just five to ten minutes each day for a simple mindfulness exercise, such as deep breathing or a brief meditation session. These small pockets of time can be woven into existing routines; perhaps during a lunch break, before sleep, or even while commuting. Additionally, technology offers tools like meditation apps that can guide a brief practice, reminding individuals to pause and refocus throughout the day. The key is to remain flexible and open-minded about how mindfulness fits into the daily schedule.

Cultivating patience and self-compassion is essential when setbacks occur on this journey. It's important to recognize that establishing a regular mindfulness practice will inevitably come with ups and downs. There may be days when distractions prevail, or when it feels impossible to quiet the mind. In these moments, practicing patience and extending self-compassion can encourage resilience. Mindfulness is not about achieving perfection but rather about being present with whatever arises, gently guiding oneself back to conscious awareness without harsh judgment. Acknowledging that setbacks are natural provides the space to continue learning and growing in the practice.

Another powerful way to address the challenges of establishing a regular mindfulness practice is by seeking community support. Engaging with others who are also practicing mindfulness can create a sense of connection and reduce feelings of isolation. This could involve joining a local mindfulness group, participating in online forums, or even sharing experiences with friends who are on a similar path.

Community support not only fosters encouragement and accountability but also enhances understanding through shared experiences. Individuals within a mindfulness community often exchange tips, resources, and encouragement, providing invaluable support and insights that enhance personal practice.

In summary, addressing common challenges in establishing a mindfulness practice involves several key elements. Identifying personal obstacles provides a clear starting point for addressing barriers. Implementing effective time management strategies allows mindfulness to seamlessly integrate into even the busiest of lives. Cultivating patience and self-compassion helps maintain commitment and resilience in the face of setbacks. Meanwhile, seeking out community support enriches the mindfulness journey through shared wisdom and encouragement. By exploring and applying these concepts, individuals can develop a sustainable and rewarding mindfulness practice that not only fits into their daily lives but also enhances their overall well-being.

Final Insights

Integrating mindfulness into daily routines can be a transformative journey, offering individuals enduring chronic pain new pathways to embrace their experiences with compassion and intention. This chapter has explored various techniques to weave mindfulness into the fabric of everyday activities, transforming ordinary moments into opportunities for presence and healing. By setting personal intentions, creating supportive environments, and finding meaning in routine tasks, you are equipped to cultivate a life that prioritizes emotional resilience and well-being. These mindful practices not only enhance your ability to manage pain but also enrich your interactions with the world around you.

As we conclude this section, it is important to reflect on the personal nature of integrating mindfulness. Each mindfulness journey is unique, tailored to individual needs and circumstances. As you continue your exploration, remember to remain patient and compassionate with yourself. Challenges may arise, but by maintaining consistency and seeking support when needed, you can foster a sustainable mindfulness practice. Through these efforts, you nurture a profound connection with your inner self, paving the way for a fulfilling and mindful existence despite the challenges chronic pain may present.

Reference List

Ainsworth, B., Atkinson, M. J., Eman AlBedah, Duncan, S., Groot, J., Jacobsen, P., James, A., Jenkins, T., Katerina Kylisova, Marks, E., Osborne, E. L., Masha Remskar, & Underhill, R. (2023, May 20). *Current Tensions and Challenges in Mindfulness Research and Practice.* https://doi.org/10.1007/s10879-023-09584-9

Banerjee, M., Cavanagh, K., & Strauss, C. (2017, November 6). *Barriers to Mindfulness: a Path Analytic Model Exploring the Role of Rumination and Worry in Predicting Psychological and Physical Engagement in an Online Mindfulness-Based Intervention.* Mindfulness. https://doi.org/10.1007/s12671-017-0837-4

Calligraphy, A. (2024, November 28). *Spiritual Mindfulness: Everyday Chores as a Path to Presence*. Medium; ILLUMINATION. https://medium.com/illumination/spiritual-mindfulness-everyday-chores-as-a-path-to-presence-cd2c246f4954

Deschene, L. (2010, July 28). *Mindfulness in Everyday Tasks: How to Get the Most from Your Chores*. Tiny Buddha. https://tinybuddha.com/blog/mindfulness-in-everyday-tasks-5-ways-chores-can-make-you-happier/

Egel, K. (2024, December 4). *Kim Egel*. Kim Egel. https://www.kimegel.com/blog/2024/12/4/mental-health-benefits-of-journaling-gaining-mindfulness-via-a-journaling-practice

How. (2024, August 5). *Calm Blog*. Calm Blog. https://www.calm.com/blog/meditation-room-ideas

Medium. (n.d.). Medium. https://coraliesawruk.medium.com/why-setting-intentions-is-the-way-to-achieve-your-goals-76d5e026d5d5

Mate, M. (2024, December 22). *Creating a Meditation Space at Home: Essentials and Inspiration*. Meditate Mate. https://mymeditatemate.com/blogs/home/creating-meditation-space-at-home-essentials-inspiration

The power of setting intentions & how to set mindful ones. (n.d.). Calm Blog. https://www.calm.com/blog/setting-intentions

allie. (2024, November 22). *Mindful Journaling: Simple Prompts for Self-Reflection and Growth*. Integrated Counseling and Wellness.

https://integratedcounselingandwellness.com/blog/mindful-journaling-simple-prompts-for-self-reflection-and-growth/

CHAPTER 5

Emotional Resilience Through Mindfulness

Emotional resilience is an invaluable ally for those dealing with chronic pain, providing a foundation to navigate the complex landscape of physical and emotional challenges that arise. In the face of ongoing discomfort, nurturing this resilience through mindfulness can create a significant shift in how individuals experience and manage their pain. As you explore the pages ahead, you'll find insights into how embracing emotions without judgment and cultivating a mindful awareness can transform daily life. This chapter invites you to embark on a journey where resilience isn't just a concept but a lived experience, offering hope and empowerment even amid difficult circumstances.

Within this exploration, the chapter delves into the intricate link between mindfulness and emotional resilience. It highlights practical strategies and exercises designed to enhance your ability to regulate emotions and cultivate compassion towards yourself. You'll discover tools that help ground you in the present moment, allowing you to view pain not as an insurmountable barrier but as a challenge that reveals strength and opportunities for growth. By incorporating practices like guided visualization and gratitude journaling into your routine, you'll be equipped to build a resilient mindset that shifts your focus from limitations to possibilities. Ultimately, this chapter serves as both a guide and a companion, supporting you as you develop the skills needed to approach chronic pain with grace and determination.

Understanding Emotional Resilience

Emotional resilience is a key asset for individuals grappling with chronic pain. It can be understood as the ability to adapt, adjust, and recover from adversity. When people face ongoing pain, emotional resilience becomes crucial. This capability allows them to manage not only physical discomfort but also the psychological strains that accompany a persistent condition. Resilient individuals often demonstrate an optimistic outlook on life, accepting pain not as a hindrance but as a part of their journey. They direct their attention inward to evaluate their emotional state, endeavoring to bolster positive emotions to mitigate pain's control over their lives (Sturgeon & Zautra, 2010). This self-awareness fosters quicker recovery and reduces negative emotions, aiding in briefer episodes of pain-induced distress.

Understanding the distinction between emotional strength and emotional suppression is essential in developing healthier strategies for coping with pain. Emotional strength involves acknowledging feelings and addressing them constructively, while suppression means ignoring or hiding emotions, which can lead to greater distress over time. An emotionally resilient person embraces their complete emotional spectrum, using both positive and negative experiences as tools for growth. Research suggests that those who express emotional complexity are better at navigating stress, showing quick recovery after negative episodes (Sturgeon & Zautra, 2013).

Several factors contribute to resilience development, including genetics, environment, and learned behaviors. Genetics may offer a baseline capacity for resilience, yet environmental influences such as supportive relationships and nurturing surroundings play a critical role in enhancing this trait. A person's immediate social network can activate and reinforce resilience resources, making interactions vital to developing resilience. Furthermore, learned behaviors like active coping and mindfulness practices can reinforce resilience by promoting engagement and reducing the perception of pain as overwhelming (Sturgeon & Zautra, 2010).

Recognizing one's personal resilience opens pathways to effectively face challenges. By appreciating their inherent strengths, individuals may feel more empowered to deal with chronic pain. This empowerment shifts their perspective, encouraging proactive approaches rather than defensive ones. Studies highlight how maintaining positive expectancies, like hope and optimism, serves as protective factors against the adverse impacts of pain, providing a buffer and fostering continued engagement despite difficulties (Sturgeon & Zautra, 2013).

A resilient mindset nurtured through these understandings transforms daily life and interactions. It supports sustainable coping mechanisms that do not just target pain relief but enhance overall life satisfaction. Individuals equipped with resilience resources like emotional knowledge and focused attention can differentiate their emotions, adapting their responses to stress effectively. These skills create opportunities for growth, enabling people to view challenges as stepping stones rather than insurmountable barriers.

The Connection Between Mindfulness and Emotional Resilience

In the journey of managing chronic pain, mindfulness offers a unique path to fostering emotional resilience. At its core, mindfulness is about cultivating an awareness and acceptance of our experiences in the present moment (Kabat-Zinn, 1994). This simple yet profound practice can be transformative when applied to the context of chronic pain and the emotional challenges that accompany it.

Mindfulness promotes awareness by encouraging individuals to observe their thoughts and emotions without judgment. This practice of attentive observation helps people become more attuned to their emotional responses. By doing so, they develop a greater understanding of their emotional landscape, which is crucial for building emotional resilience. Instead of being swept away by waves of fear or anxiety triggered by pain, mindfulness helps individuals stand grounded, observing these emotions as transient moments rather than permanent states. This heightened awareness allows for better emotional regulation, contributing to resilience in the face of pain (Keng et al., 2011).

Acceptance, another cornerstone of mindfulness, plays a vital role in enhancing emotional resilience. Often, the instinctive reaction to pain is resistance, which can intensify suffering. Mindfulness teaches acceptance of whatever arises in the present moment, including discomfort and negative emotions. Accepting these experiences without trying to change them diminishes their power and reduces psychological distress (Oh et al., 2022). It opens up space for compassion toward oneself during painful episodes, fostering a gentle attitude that strengthens emotional resilience over time.

One of the significant benefits of engaging in mindfulness practices is the ability to reframe negative thought patterns. Chronic pain often comes with a barrage of negative thoughts—doubts about recovery, fears of worsening conditions, or frustrations over perceived limitations. Through mindful awareness, individuals learn to recognize and challenge these destructive thought patterns, viewing them as mental constructs rather than truths. This cognitive reframing is crucial in reducing the emotional weight of pain, allowing individuals to approach their condition with a more balanced perspective.

Mindfulness also nurtures a compassionate response to pain instead of succumbing to fear or frustration. By practicing self-compassion, individuals learn to treat themselves with kindness, much like they would a friend experiencing similar struggles. Rather than judging themselves harshly for their limitations or setbacks, they respond with understanding and empathy. This shift from self-criticism to self-compassion not only eases emotional suffering but also bolsters resilience by fostering a nurturing inner dialogue (Hanh, 1976).

Building mindfulness habits is integral to establishing a foundation for lasting emotional resilience. Introducing mindfulness into daily routines creates a continuous thread of awareness throughout one's life. Whether through formal meditation practices, mindful breathing exercises, or simply taking moments to pause and reflect, these habits deepen resilience by reinforcing the skills of awareness, acceptance, and compassion. Over time, individuals find themselves better equipped to handle the unpredictable nature of chronic pain, responding with composure rather than overwhelm (Oh et al., 2022).

While it might seem daunting to incorporate mindfulness into an already challenging life, it's important to remember that this practice doesn't have to be complex. Starting small, perhaps with a few minutes of conscious breathing each day, can lay the groundwork for deeper exploration. Gradually increasing mindfulness activities as comfort levels rise ensures sustainable integration into daily life.

For those beginning their mindfulness journey, guided programs like Mindfulness-Based Stress Reduction (MBSR) offer structured pathways to developing these skills. MBSR provides tools to relate to physical and emotional experiences more openly and nonjudgmentally, facilitating personal growth in handling chronic pain (Kabat-Zinn, 1982). Participants often report a shift in their relationship with pain—from antagonistic to accepting—fostering resilience as they navigate the ups and downs of their condition.

Mindfulness in Enhancing Emotional Awareness

Mindfulness offers a pathway to enhancing emotional awareness and resilience, particularly for individuals dealing with chronic pain. By developing an acute understanding of one's emotions, sufferers can identify triggers that exacerbate their pain. Emotional awareness enables individuals to discern the nuanced interplay between their feelings and physical experiences. Recognizing patterns in feelings such as stress, anxiety, or fear that magnify pain empowers individuals to address these triggers effectively. For instance, someone may notice that tension builds up before a flare-up, allowing them to adopt proactive measures like relaxation techniques to mitigate pain.

Journaling is a specific mindfulness technique that fosters emotional reflection, enabling people to uncover the deeper implications of their emotional states on pain levels. Through the act of writing down thoughts and feelings, individuals can gain clarity and perspective on their emotional experiences. This practice facilitates a better understanding of how certain emotions influence pain perceptions and allows for the development of strategies to manage them. As described by Wright (2023), journaling aids in processing complex emotions, offering a structured way to articulate feelings and assess their origins. It serves not just as a record but as a tool for introspection, providing insights that help adjust responses to both emotional and physical challenges.

Acceptance, a core tenet of mindfulness, plays a pivotal role in diminishing resistance to pain and cultivating healthier emotional responses. When individuals approach their pain with acceptance rather than resistance, they reduce the psychological burden associated with continual struggle. According to Keng et al. (2011), mindfulness encourages a nonjudgmental acceptance of one's moment-to-moment experience, reducing tendencies to avoid or suppress discomforting thoughts and emotions. This shift from resistance to acceptance changes how pain is perceived, transforming it into something manageable rather than overwhelming. Acceptance also promotes emotional liberation, as individuals learn to coexist with their feelings without letting them dictate their lives.

Increased emotional intelligence derived from mindfulness becomes a crucial asset in facilitating better communication with healthcare providers. Enhanced awareness and articulation of one's emotional and physical state lead to more productive interactions during medical consultations. Patients can convey their symptoms and emotional concerns more accurately, encouraging collaborative efforts in pain management strategies. By fostering open and clear communication, patients become active participants in their healthcare journeys, which can result in more tailored and effective treatment plans.

Practical mindfulness exercises can be integrated seamlessly into daily routines to bolster emotional resilience. Techniques such as deep breathing, guided visualization, and mindful body scans offer immediate benefits by grounding individuals in the present moment. These practices train attention and foster a sense of calm, aiding in the regulation of emotional responses to pain. By dedicating even a few minutes each day to mindfulness exercises, individuals can build a mental toolkit that strengthens their emotional foundations and prepares them to handle fluctuations in pain and mood more effectively.

Setting resilience goals ensures that mindfulness practices remain focused and purposeful. Goals should be specific, measurable, achievable, relevant, and time-bound (SMART criteria) to guide personal growth. When individuals set clear intentions for their mindfulness journey—such as dedicating ten minutes daily to meditation—they create a structured path towards enhanced emotional resilience. Tracking progress towards these goals cultivates a sense of accomplishment and motivates continued engagement with mindfulness practices.

Creating a supportive environment also enhances the effectiveness of mindfulness practices in building resilience. Engaging in mindfulness within communities—whether through group meditation sessions or discussions about emotional experiences—fosters a sense of belonging and shared purpose. Open dialogues about mindfulness and its benefits encourage collective growth, while designated mindfulness spaces provide a safe haven for individual practice. By surrounding oneself with a nurturing environment, individuals reinforce their commitment to emotional health and well-being.

Lastly, regular reflection and adjustment of mindfulness practices ensure that they remain relevant to one's evolving needs. Chronic pain conditions can fluctuate, necessitating adaptable approaches to mindfulness. Periodically reassessing goals, techniques, and outcomes allows individuals to fine-tune their practices to align with current circumstances. Whether it's incorporating new mindfulness exercises or revisiting foundational practices, maintaining flexibility in one's approach guarantees continued progress in emotional resilience.

Building Resilience Strategies Through Mindfulness

Mindfulness and resilience are powerful partners in empowering individuals to manage chronic pain more effectively. By integrating mindfulness practices with resilience-building techniques, individuals can cultivate a robust toolkit to navigate their pain experiences. Let's explore some practical strategies and exercises that foster emotional resilience through mindfulness.

One of the cornerstone mindfulness exercises that bolster resilience is guided visualization. This practice involves closing your eyes and envisioning a place where you feel completely at ease—a peaceful beach, a serene forest, or any space that evokes calm. As you immerse yourself in this mental imagery, notice the sensations, sounds, and scents around you. This exercise not only provides a temporary escape from physical discomfort but also strengthens your ability to manage stress by inviting a sense of tranquility into your daily life. It serves as a mental rehearsal that enhances resilience by reinforcing your capacity to return to a state of calm amidst pain.

Gratitude practices are another mindfulness technique that significantly contributes to building resilience. Keeping a gratitude journal, for instance, encourages you to jot down a few things you are grateful for each day. It shifts focus from pain to positive experiences, instilling hope and enhancing emotional strength. Over time, this shift in focus helps rewire the brain to recognize and embrace positivity, which lays the foundation for greater resilience against the challenges posed by chronic pain.

Establishing clear resilience goals isn't just about wishful thinking; it's about setting actionable and realistic objectives using SMART criteria—Specific, Measurable, Achievable, Relevant, and Time-bound. For example, a goal might be to engage in a five-minute mindfulness meditation every morning for two weeks. Specificity keeps you focused, measurability allows tracking progress, achievability ensures that you're setting realistic targets, relevance aligns goals with personal values, and time-bounding creates urgency. This structured approach promotes personal growth efficiently, allowing you to see tangible improvements in your resilience over time (Cothran & Wysocki, 2019).

Creating supportive environments plays a critical role in enhancing resilience. Open dialogue within these environments fosters a sense of safety and understanding. Engaging in conversations about challenges and victories with loved ones or support groups encourages mutual support and shared learning. Additionally, establishing mindfulness spaces at home or in community settings can provide a sanctuary for practice and reflection. These spaces, free from judgment and distraction, enable you to cultivate mindfulness routines that strengthen resilience.

Continuous reflection on resilience strategies is vital, especially when dealing with fluctuating pain levels. Regularly assessing what strategies are effective allows for adaptation and relevancy in managing pain. This could involve keeping a reflective journal where you note how different approaches impact your emotional state and resilience. Reflective practices encourage an ongoing process of learning and adaptation, reinforcing the importance of being tuned into one's emotional landscape. This adaptability enables you to adjust your strategies to align with current needs, ensuring that your resilience mechanisms remain relevant and effective (Rose, 2024).

Incorporating these mindfulness and resilience-building strategies requires commitment, but the payoffs are significant. Mindfulness practices such as guided visualization and gratitude journaling cultivate a mindset shift that strengthens emotional resilience. Establishing resilience goals using SMART criteria ensures that your efforts are directed towards meaningful growth. Supportive environments and continuous reflection further reinforce your resilience journey, equipping you with the tools needed to face chronic pain with courage and calm.

Impact of Mindfulness and Resilience on Emotional Health

In the realm of chronic pain management, emotional resilience emerges as a beacon of hope. Mindfulness offers tangible benefits in this quest by weaving together improved emotion regulation and boosting overall emotional health. When confronted with chronic pain, emotions often become intense and overwhelming. This is where mindfulness steps in, fostering a balanced emotional landscape that helps individuals navigate their experiences more adeptly.

Studies have consistently shown that mindfulness enhances one's ability to regulate emotions, allowing individuals to observe their feelings without immediate reaction or judgment (Keng et al., 2011). By cultivating this mindful awareness, people can develop a better understanding of their emotional responses, thereby reducing the likelihood of being swept away by negative emotions like anxiety and frustration, which are common companions of chronic pain. With regular mindfulness practice, one learns to embrace emotions, observing them with curiosity rather than fear or avoidance. This shift paves the way for healthier emotional processing, encouraging a state of peace even amidst turmoil.

Furthermore, mindfulness offers powerful adaptive coping strategies that mitigate emotional distress and improve response to pain flare-ups. These strategies include techniques such as focused breathing, body scans, and meditation. Adopting these coping mechanisms allows for a more grounded response to stressors, enhancing one's ability to manage pain-induced emotional upheavals. For example, integrating mindfulness meditation into daily life has been shown to reduce symptoms like depression and anxiety while promoting a positive outlook on life (Oh et al., 2022). This not only eases the burden of pain but also equips individuals with tools to approach future challenges with poise and confidence.

A resilient mindset nurtured through mindfulness transforms perspectives on pain, creating a sense of empowerment. Instead of viewing pain solely as an adversary, individuals may begin to perceive it as a teacher, offering lessons in patience, strength, and adaptability. This empowered viewpoint catalyzes personal growth, shifting the narrative from victimhood to agency. By embracing this resilient mindset, individuals gain the fortitude to face adversity head-on, transforming their experience of pain from one of suffering to one of resilience and strength.

Mindfulness and resilience collectively enhance emotional well-being, contributing substantially to greater life satisfaction. Living with chronic pain can often feel like an uphill battle, but when equipped with the tools of mindfulness, individuals find moments of joy and contentment within their reach. Regular mindfulness practice encourages a shift in focus from pain to gratitude, emphasizing what is present and valuable in one's life. This shift fosters a deep appreciation for life's small pleasures, nurturing satisfaction and happiness even amidst ongoing challenges. As mindfulness becomes ingrained in daily routines, the ripple effect manifests in improved relationships, increased engagement in activities, and a profound sense of inner peace.

Guidelines for incorporating mindfulness into daily life can serve as a roadmap towards enhanced emotional resilience. Simple practices, such as setting aside time for quiet reflection or engaging in mindful walking, offer opportunities to ground oneself in the present moment. Journaling can also be a valuable tool, providing space to explore emotions and monitor progress over time. By integrating these practices into everyday life, individuals cultivate a rich foundation of mindfulness that supports resilience during trying times.

Concluding Thoughts

As we journey through the insights of this chapter, we've explored how building emotional resilience plays a pivotal role in coping with chronic pain. Embracing mindfulness as a tool invites us to delve deeper into our emotions, turning them from turbulent waters into calm streams that flow gently through the landscape of our minds. By acknowledging and accepting our feelings without judgment, we learn to navigate the complexities of our emotional responses. This understanding grants us the strength to transform pain from a formidable adversary into a manageable travel companion on our path to healing.

Mindfulness not only sharpens our awareness but also nurtures a compassionate relationship with ourselves, fostering kindness over harsh self-criticism. Simple practices like guided visualization invite serenity, while gratitude journaling shifts focus towards positivity. These steps build a resilient framework that allows for growth, seen less as a struggle and more as an evolution. As you incorporate these mindfulness strategies into your daily routine, you may find yourself better equipped to face life's challenges with courage and grace, discovering moments of joy even amidst the shadows of pain.

Reference List

Keng, S. L., Smoski, M. J., & Robins, C. J. (2011). *Effects of Mindfulness on Psychological health: a Review of Empirical Studies.* Clinical Psychology Review. https://doi.org/10.1016/j.cpr.2011.04.006

Oh, V. K. S., Sarwar, A., & Pervez, N. (2022, December 21). *The study of mindfulness as an intervening factor for enhanced psychological well-being in building the level of resilience.* Figshare.com. https://doi.org/10.3389/fpsyg.2022.1056834

Rose, M. (2024, June 10). *Self-help Strategies: Rose Behavioral Health's Guide to Personal Wellness - Rose Behavioral Health.* Rose Behavioral Health. https://www.rosebehavioralhealth.com/self-help-strategies-rose-behavioral-healths-guide-to-personal-wellness/

Riopel, L. (2019, April 10). *Goal Setting in Counseling and Therapy (Incl. Workbooks & Templates).* PositivePsychology.com. https://positivepsychology.com/goal-setting-counseling-therapy/

Sturgeon, J. A., & Zautra, A. J. (2010, March 2). *Resilience: A New Paradigm for Adaptation to Chronic Pain.* Current Pain and Headache Reports. https://doi.org/10.1007/s11916-010-0095-9

Sturgeon, J. A., & Zautra, A. J. (2013, January 22). *Psychological Resilience, Pain Catastrophizing, and Positive Emotions: Perspectives on Comprehensive Modeling of Individual Pain Adaptation.* Current Pain and Headache Reports. https://doi.org/10.1007/s11916-012-0317-4

Wright, K. W. (2023, June 21). *Emotional journaling: How to use journaling to process emotions*. Day One. https://dayoneapp.com/blog/emotional-journaling/

CHAPTER 6

Pain Perception and the Mind-Body Connection

Pain perception and the mind-body connection are intricate aspects of the human experience, ripe for exploration. Pain is not just a physical sensation; it weaves through our emotions, thoughts, and behaviors, influencing every facet of daily life. For those dealing with chronic pain, understanding how the mind and body interact can be transformative, offering new ways to cope and heal. Mindfulness practices stand out as a bridge, connecting the mental and physical realms in a compassionate dialogue. These techniques encourage individuals to become more aware of their inner experiences, promoting a shift from reacting to pain to observing it with curiosity and acceptance. This perspective opens up opportunities for healing that address both the mind and body, creating a path forward with empathy and self-care.

In this chapter, you'll delve into the profound impact mindfulness has on altering pain perception and enhancing the mind-body connection. We will examine how historical approaches to pain management often overlooked the psychological components, focusing predominantly on physical symptoms. Through an empathetic lens, we explore how modern research recognizes pain as a complex experience shaped by sensory, emotional, and cognitive dimensions. By incorporating mindfulness practices such as meditation and focused breathing exercises, you'll discover how individuals can alter their pain experiences, fostering resilience and reducing anxiety. The chapter presents practical strategies, supported by scientific insights, to empower those living with chronic pain, guiding them towards a deeper understanding of themselves and their path to well-being.

Mind-Body Dualism

The concept of mind-body dualism has long fascinated scholars, tracing back to the philosophical musings of René Descartes. This theory posits a distinct separation between the mental and physical realms, suggesting that the mind and body function independently of one another. Historically, this separation has influenced medical approaches, often prioritizing the treatment of physical symptoms while neglecting the significant role the mind plays in pain perception. This distinction has sometimes led to an oversight where the psychological components of pain are not adequately addressed, leaving individuals with chronic pain feeling misunderstood and inadequately treated (Namjoo et al., 2019).

In traditional views, the separation of mind and body was stark, with each aspect given individual attention. However, contemporary scientific insights reveal the importance of integrating mental states into the understanding of physical pain. Modern research emphasizes that pain is not merely a physical phenomenon but a complex experience influenced by cognitive and emotional processes. The recognition of pain as multifaceted—comprising sensory, emotional, and cognitive dimensions—opens the door to more comprehensive management strategies that effectively address both mind and body (Cosio & Sujata Swaroop, 2016). Mindfulness emerges as a pivotal practice in bridging the gap within this dualistic framework.

Mindfulness practices encourage individuals to become more attuned to their thoughts and bodily sensations. By fostering a state of self-awareness, mindfulness allows patients to perceive pain differently. Rather than viewing pain solely as a negative and overpowering force, mindfulness encourages a non-judgmental approach that acknowledges pain's presence without letting it dominate one's entire existence. This shift in perspective can significantly alter how individuals experience and react to pain, promoting acceptance and reducing anxiety related to chronic pain conditions (Namjoo et al., 2019).

Integrating mindfulness into pain management introduces a unique opportunity to unite the mind and body in the healing process. When individuals engage in mindfulness practices, such as meditation or focused breathing exercises, they learn to observe their pain without immediate reaction or fear. This practice nurtures a sense of detachment, where pain is recognized as a transient sensation rather than an insurmountable obstacle. Through regular mindfulness exercises, patients develop greater resilience against the mental toll of chronic pain, consequently diminishing the intensity and impact of their pain experiences (Cosio & Sujata Swaroop, 2016).

An empathetic consideration of the mind-body connection recognizes that the interplay between mental and physical states is central to comprehending pain. Mindfulness stands as a bridge that unites these two seemingly disparate elements, providing a holistic approach to pain management. As patients engage in mindfulness, they cultivate an environment where the mind and body coexist harmoniously, fostering healing and enhancing overall well-being. This integration underscores the potential for mindfulness to transform traditional pain management paradigms and offer new pathways for relief (Namjoo et al., 2019).

Mindfulness practices, like mindful meditation and body scans, activate neural pathways linked to attention and emotion regulation, offering empirical support for the efficacy of integrating mindfulness in pain management. By consistently practicing these techniques, individuals can tap into the mind's power to modulate pain perception. This modulation occurs as mindfulness helps restructure how pain is processed in the brain, creating an adaptive cognitive and emotional environment within which pain is perceived less intensely (Cosio & Sujata Swaroop, 2016).

Moreover, mindfulness fosters a mindset of openness and acceptance, essential qualities for managing chronic pain. As patients embrace non-judgmental observation, they reduce the burden of intrusive negative thoughts and emotions that often accompany chronic pain conditions. Through this practice, patients experience less stress and anxiety, as mindfulness teaches them to focus on the present moment, freeing them from anticipatory dread and rumination over past pain episodes. Such a transformation in mindset enables individuals to live more meaningful, less pain-dominated lives (Namjoo et al., 2019).

Role of Perception in Pain

Pain perception is a nuanced experience, often misunderstood as a direct result of physical harm. But it's vital to recognize that psychological factors and interpretations play a monumental role in shaping how we perceive pain. Cognitive and mindfulness techniques can alter the intensity of our pain experiences by influencing these factors.

Studies reveal that cognitive frameworks deeply affect our pain perception. Our thoughts and emotions can amplify or diminish sensations, showcasing the mind's power over bodily experiences (Apkarian et al., 2011). When we direct attention away from pain, its intensity may decrease, reflecting the intricate relationship between thought processes and sensory perceptions (Bantick et al., 2002). Mindfulness, in particular, encourages observing thoughts without attachment, allowing for a shift in the way we experience pain.

Mindfulness offers a powerful means of transforming pain experiences. Rooted in an ancient tradition, it involves maintaining awareness of the present moment with acceptance and non-judgment (Kabat-Zinn, 2003). This mental state empowers individuals to revisit painful stimuli with equanimity, thereby promoting better acceptance and reducing reactive responses (Hayes et al., 1999). Instead of attempting to avoid or alter uncomfortable sensations, mindfulness teaches individuals to acknowledge these experiences with a calm, undisturbed mindset (Lu et al., 2023).

Real-life case studies highlight noticeable changes in pain perception through mindfulness, emphasizing the significant impact such practices can have on one's quality of life. A landmark study observed mindfulness experts reporting lower pain when focusing their attention on the pain site compared to novices (Gard et al., 2012). These differences underscore how trained mindfulness practitioners can successfully recast their pain experiences through focused attention and nonjudgmental awareness.

Furthermore, mindfulness techniques like breath focus and sensory awareness are pivotal tools in easing suffering. By anchoring attention to the breath, individuals can cultivate a sense of stability and centeredness amidst pain, simplifying complex sensations into manageable experiences. Sensory awareness, on the other hand, helps precisely identify pain triggers and patterns, facilitating more informed interactions with bodily sensations (Zeidan et al., 2012). Such mindful approaches create space between perception and reaction, significantly recasting pain.

Contrary to popular belief, pain is not solely a physical phenomenon. It is constructed from an interaction of sensory, cognitive, and emotional processes (Zeidan et al., 2012). The modulation of pain through mindfulness capitalizes on this interaction, demonstrating that perception significantly influences the subjective experience of pain. For chronic pain sufferers, this insight holds promise for novel management strategies aimed at improving life quality.

Beyond theoretical evidence, practical applications further demonstrate mindfulness's potential. Integrating mindfulness into daily routines provides a sustainable path for pain management, addressing both immediate discomfort and long-term health. Mindful attitudes and attentiveness work symbiotically to fortify resilience against pain's grip (Duan, 2014). As individuals become adept at non-reactive observation, they foster an accepting attitude that can fundamentally alter pain-related fear learning, leading to relief and empowerment (Taylor et al., 2018).

The transformative potential of mindfulness is most apparent in its ability to teach individuals to perceive pain differently. Instead of merely enduring pain, people learn to engage with it constructively. Through regular practice, mindfulness fosters self-awareness and nonjudgmental observation, reducing anxiety and tension linked to chronic pain conditions. By shifting the internal narrative around pain, sufferers can gain new perspectives that redefine their relationship with discomfort (Martinez-Calderon et al., 2019).

While mindfulness presents an alternative strategy for managing chronic pain, it does so without negating the reality of physical sensations. Rather, it invites a holistic view that integrates psychological dimensions into understanding pain. As supported by extensive research, mindfulness stands as a promising approach that aligns with modern insights into the mind-body connection, all while empowering individuals to regain control over their pain experiences.

Enhancing Sensory Awareness

Enhancing sensory awareness through mindfulness plays a pivotal role in improving pain management by engaging individuals more deeply with their bodily sensations. This engagement allows them to develop a more nuanced understanding of their pain, unveiling specific triggers and patterns that might otherwise remain hidden. By becoming attuned to these experiences, individuals can start to decipher the language of their bodies, thereby altering the way pain is perceived.

Mindfulness techniques such as body scans and mindful walking are particularly beneficial in fostering this heightened state of bodily engagement. During a body scan meditation, for instance, practitioners lie down and focus their attention on different parts of their body, from toes to head, consciously noting any sensations, emotions, or thoughts linked to each area (Mayo Clinic Staff, 2022). Similarly, mindful walking encourages individuals to focus on the experience of movement, paying attention to each step and the sensations associated with standing and balancing. Such practices cultivate a deeper connection between mind and body, promoting positive pain experiences by increasing sensory awareness and reducing the tendency to react negatively to discomfort.

Studies corroborate these observations by linking mindfulness-induced sensory awareness to decreased pain sensitivity. Neuroimaging research has demonstrated that mindfulness engages brain regions involved in sensory processing and pain modulation. The activation of areas such as the right anterior insula and the orbitofrontal cortex supports the notion that mindfulness enhances one's ability to modulate sensory input, leading to reductions in pain intensity and unpleasantness (Zeidan & Vago, 2016). These findings underline the potential of mindfulness not merely as a passive coping mechanism but as an active intervention that influences the neural pathways associated with pain perception.

For individuals suffering from chronic pain, practical exercises centered around daily mindfulness can be transformative. Establishing new relationships with pain involves inviting a sense of curiosity and observation instead of judgment. Whether it's through guided imagery, focusing on breath, or savoring sensory experiences like the taste and smell of food, mindfulness exercises encourage individuals to live fully in the moment. This approach not only helps manage pain but also fosters a sense of empowerment and control over one's experiences.

A guideline here would be empowering patients to take control of their pain experience through mindfulness practices.

Practicing mindfulness consistently, perhaps starting with short, manageable sessions and gradually extending the duration, is key to gaining its full benefits. The aim is to make mindfulness a regular part of one's routine, potentially integrating it into everyday activities. This might involve dedicating time early in the morning for structured exercises, allowing for introspective moments free from distraction (Mayo Clinic Staff, 2022).

Mindfulness and Neuroplasticity

Pain perception is a deeply personal experience, shaped by mental factors and, intriguingly, our brain's ability to change. This adaptability is known as neuroplasticity, which refers to the brain's capacity to reorganize itself by forming new neural connections. Neuroplasticity is particularly significant in the context of pain because it suggests that the way we perceive pain can be altered through our experiences and practices.

Mindfulness is an influential tool in this reorganization process. Practicing mindfulness can affect how our brain manages and interprets pain. With ongoing research, scientists have identified changes in brain structures involved in pain regulation attributable to mindfulness practices. Studies indicate that mindfulness enhances gray matter density in areas connected to pain processing (Zeidan et al., 2019). This physical alteration within the brain demonstrates that consistent mindfulness training can lead to tangible physiological changes that influence pain perception.

Chronic pain often leads to maladaptive changes in the brain. These are negative developments that can worsen one's pain experience over time. However, engaging regularly in mindfulness practices can counteract these adverse effects by promoting positive neural adaptations. Through mindfulness, individuals can foster beneficial changes in their brain's structure that help alleviate chronic pain symptoms (Zeidan & Vago, 2016).

Various forms of mindfulness, such as meditation and focused breathing exercises, are particularly effective in supporting neuroplasticity for those dealing with chronic pain. Mindfulness-based interventions like the Mindfulness-Based Stress Reduction (MBSR) program have been shown to improve pain symptoms and overall quality of life for participants. In fact, the MBSR has spawned extensive research initiatives focused on its impact on chronic pain management (Kabat-Zinn et al., 56).

Importantly, the benefits of mindfulness on neuroplasticity and pain relief underscore the need for a proactive approach to incorporating mindfulness techniques into daily routines. By doing so, individuals can cultivate an environment conducive to continual healing and adaptation. Consistency in practice allows the brain to strengthen its newly formed pathways, promoting lasting changes in how pain is perceived and managed.

For someone experiencing chronic pain, implementing mindfulness practices provides a pathway to developing heightened self-awareness. This newfound awareness encourages individuals to delve deeply into their pain experiences, gaining insights that might otherwise go unnoticed. Creating a space where one can observe pain without judgment fosters an understanding that can alter how pain is perceived and processed.

Keep the mind present. Mindfulness enhances the ability to focus on the present moment, which can significantly reduce fear and anxiety associated with chronic pain. In doing so, individuals may find relief from the anticipatory dread that often accompanies persistent discomfort. The practice of staying grounded in the here-and-now shifts attention away from pain's distressing aspects, thereby altering its emotional impact (Zeidan et al., 2019).

The cumulative result of integrating mindfulness practices lies not just in temporary relief but in long-term gains in reshaping one's experience of pain. Mindfulness techniques encourage people to engage actively with their healing journey, nurturing a sense of empowerment and control over their condition. As these techniques become woven into everyday life, they serve as a steadfast companion in the endeavor to transform pain from a debilitating force into a manageable part of life.

Influence of Thoughts on Pain

Pain perception is deeply intertwined with the mind-body connection, where our thoughts and emotions heavily influence how we experience pain. Negative thought patterns can substantially escalate one's perception of pain, making it feel more intense than its actual physical cause might suggest. Mindfulness offers a unique approach to this challenge by encouraging individuals to observe their thoughts without judgment, allowing for a shift in perspective that can significantly alter one's pain experience (Wasson et al., 2020).

The power of cognitive-behavioral strategies combined with mindfulness is seen in their ability to transform narratives around pain. By restructuring these narratives, patients can find new ways to interpret and manage their pain experiences.

Cognitive-behavioral therapy (CBT) has been widely recognized for its efficacy in managing chronic pain through techniques that decrease catastrophizing—an exaggerated negative orientation towards pain—and increase self-efficacy (Turner et al., 2016). These techniques aim to change how patients perceive their pain, promoting a sense of control over their experiences.

Mindfulness practices, when integrated into CBT, create an even more powerful tool for reshaping pain experiences. These practices focus on being present and acknowledging thoughts and sensations without immediate reaction or attachment. This non-judgmental observation helps cultivate self-compassion, acceptance, and gratitude, which are positively correlated with better pain management outcomes. It's about shifting from a reactive state to a responsive one, where recognizing thoughts as merely thoughts, rather than facts, can reduce stress and anxiety associated with pain.

Practical strategies for integrating mindfulness into daily life can include keeping thought diaries. These diaries allow individuals to track recurring negative thoughts related to pain and analyze them with a mindful lens. This practice not only highlights unhealthy patterns but also provides opportunities to reframe these thoughts constructively. For example, a person might realize they often feel "this pain will never go away," which could be reframed as "this moment is difficult, but I have managed similar moments before."

Mindfulness also proves beneficial during overwhelming moments when pain seems all-consuming. Simple exercises, such as deep breathing or brief meditation sessions, can promote calmness and recentering. Additionally, collaborating with healthcare providers to develop consistent mental strategies ensures individuals receive personalized support, enhancing the effectiveness of mindfulness practices. When healthcare providers and patients work together, they can tailor these strategies to best fit individual needs, ensuring long-term adherence and success.

Understanding that pain is influenced by psychological factors, not just physical injury, underscores the importance of addressing the mind's role in pain management. Through mindfulness, individuals learn to recognize and gradually accept their pain without letting it define them. In doing so, they foster resilience and compassion towards themselves, reducing the emotional burden that often accompanies chronic pain.

Perception plays a crucial role in pain experiences, allowing for varying intensities based on individual interpretation. When perception is manipulated through mindfulness and cognitive techniques, it becomes possible to lessen the grip pain holds over one's life. Mindfulness empowers individuals by making them aware of these perceptions, enabling them to choose how they engage with pain rather than feeling overwhelmed by it.

Summary and Reflections

This chapter has cast light on the profound link between mindfulness and pain perception, inviting us to rethink how we view the relationship between the mind and body. By exploring this connection, we recognize that pain is not just a physical sensation but a complex interplay of emotions, thoughts, and beliefs. Mindfulness acts as a gentle guide, steering individuals away from fear and towards a place of acceptance and understanding. This shift in perspective allows for a more compassionate interaction with one's own body, helping to reduce the intensity of pain while promoting emotional resilience.

As we've seen, embracing mindfulness can lead to remarkable changes in how pain is experienced. It empowers individuals to pay close attention to their sensations without letting them dictate their lives. Through practices like meditation, deep breathing, and mindful observation, people learn to detach from overwhelming pain and discover inner peace. This journey towards heightened awareness not only transforms the way pain is managed but also fosters a sense of empowerment and control. Ultimately, by integrating mindfulness into daily life, one cultivates a nurturing environment where healing becomes attainable and holistic well-being is within reach.

Reference List

Cosio, D., & Sujata Swaroop. (2016, March 30). *The Use of Mind-body Medicine in Chronic Pain Management: Differential Trends and Session-by-Session Changes in Anxiety.* Journal of Pain Management & Medicine. https://pmc.ncbi.nlm.nih.gov/articles/PMC4855874/

Lu, C., Moliadze, V., & Nees, F. (2023, November 9). *Dynamic processes of mindfulness-based alterations in pain perception.* Frontiers in Neuroscience; Frontiers Media. https://doi.org/10.3389/fnins.2023.1253559

Mayo Clinic Staff. (2022, October 11). *Mindfulness exercises.* Mayo Clinic. https://www.mayoclinic.org/healthy-lifestyle/consumer-health/in-depth/mindfulness-exercises/art-20046356

Namjoo, S., Borjali, A., Seirafi, M., & Assarzadegan, F. (2019, October 20). *Use of Mindfulness-based Cognitive Therapy to Change Pain-related Cognitive Processing in Patients with Primary Headache: A Randomized Trial with Attention Placebo Control Group.* Anesthesiology and Pain Medicine. https://doi.org/10.5812/aapm.91927

Turner, J. A., Anderson, M. L., Balderson, B. H., Cook, A. J., Sherman, K. J., & Cherkin, D. C. (2016, November). *Mindfulness-based stress reduction and cognitive behavioral therapy for chronic low back pain.* PAIN. https://doi.org/10.1097/j.pain.0000000000000635

Wasson, R. S., Barratt, C., & O'Brien, W. H. (2020, March 5). *Effects of Mindfulness-Based Interventions on Self-compassion in Health Care Professionals: a Meta-analysis.* Mindfulness. https://doi.org/10.1007/s12671-020-01342-5

Zeidan, F., & Vago, D. R. (2016, June). *Mindfulness meditation-based pain relief: a mechanistic account.* Annals of the New York Academy of Sciences. https://doi.org/10.1111/nyas.13153

Zeidan, F., Grant, J. A., Brown, C. A., McHaffie, J. G., & Coghill, R. C. (2012, June). *Mindfulness meditation-related pain relief: Evidence for unique brain mechanisms in the regulation of pain.* Neuroscience Letters. https://doi.org/10.1016/j.neulet.2012.03.082

Zeidan, F., Baumgartner, J. N., & Coghill, R. C. (2019). *The neural mechanisms of mindfulness-based pain relief.* PAIN Reports. https://doi.org/10.1097/pr9.0000000000000759

CHAPTER 7

Mindfulness-Based Stress Reduction

Mindfulness-Based Stress Reduction (MBSR) offers an innovative approach to managing stress and pain through mindfulness practices. Emerging from the creative vision of Dr. Jon Kabat-Zinn in the 1970s, MBSR initially addressed a critical gap in healthcare: providing relief for those with chronic illnesses that did not fully respond to traditional treatments. Its blend of mindfulness meditation, yoga, and body awareness techniques invites individuals on a journey to engage deeply with their experiences. This revolutionary program empowers participants by transforming how they perceive and manage stressors, fostering a sense of agency in their healing process.

In this chapter, you will embark on an exploration of MBSR's evolution from its foundational roots to its widespread application in various sectors such as healthcare, education, and business. Discover how MBSR's core principles—non-judgment, acceptance, and body awareness—can reshape one's relationship with pain and stress. We'll delve into different techniques like mindful meditation, body scanning, and mindful walking that are central to MBSR's effectiveness. You'll also learn about the supportive community aspect of MBSR that enhances personal growth and resilience. Through a combination of scientific evidence and personal narratives, this chapter unfolds the transformative potential of MBSR for improving mental well-being and quality of life for those seeking alternative therapeutic paths.

History of MBSR

In the late 1970s, Dr. Jon Kabat-Zinn developed Mindfulness-Based Stress Reduction (MBSR) as a response to the increasing need for non-traditional therapeutic practices. At the time, many individuals struggled with chronic illnesses such as stress and pain but found limited relief through conventional medicine. Recognizing this gap, Dr. Kabat-Zinn introduced MBSR as a revolutionary approach that incorporated mindfulness meditation, yoga, and body awareness techniques to help people manage stress and pain more effectively.

The initial application of MBSR was in medical settings where it quickly demonstrated its transformative role in healthcare. The program was designed to serve patients experiencing chronic pain, depression, anxiety, and other stress-related conditions. This innovative method encouraged individuals to engage with their experiences directly and mindfully, enhancing their ability to cope with symptoms that traditional treatments couldn't fully address. As a result, MBSR gained traction among healthcare practitioners who were searching for complementary interventions that offered tangible benefits without the side effects commonly associated with pharmaceuticals.

One of MBSR's most significant contributions to healthcare is its ability to complement conventional treatments. Unlike some alternative therapies, which could be seen as conflicting with standard medical practices, MBSR works in harmony with them. By fostering greater awareness and acceptance of present-moment experiences, MBSR empowers patients to participate actively in their healing process. This empowerment can lead to improved patient outcomes, as individuals learn to navigate their physical and emotional challenges more skillfully. The reduction of stress levels can also promote better overall health, making MBSR an appealing option for integration into various medical disciplines.

Over the years, MBSR has evolved to meet the needs of diverse populations, highlighting its flexibility and continued relevance on a global scale. Initially, the focus was primarily on addressing chronic pain and stress within clinical environments. Yet, as the program's effectiveness became evident, it expanded beyond hospitals and clinics to reach schools, workplaces, and communities worldwide. This growth was driven by the recognition that stress and pain are universal experiences that transcend cultural and demographic boundaries. Thus, adapting MBSR to suit the unique needs of different groups became essential.

Today, MBSR is offered in over 720 medical centers and clinics across the globe, reflecting its widespread acceptance and implementation ([*History of MBSR*, n.d.]). The program has also inspired similar initiatives aimed at integrating mindfulness into mainstream institutions like education, business, sports, and even prisons. This far-reaching impact showcases MBSR's adaptability and underscores its enduring relevance in modern society. The program's success lies not only in its therapeutic potential but also in its capacity to instill values of mindfulness and compassion within individuals and communities alike.

A key aspect of MBSR's evolution has been its ability to adapt its techniques to fit the contexts and needs of various populations. For instance, individuals with chronic illnesses such as diabetes, hypertension, cancer, and immune disorders have benefited from MBSR due to its low-risk nature and emphasis on self-regulation ([Niazi & Niazi, 2011]). By equipping patients with mindful awareness tools, MBSR helps reduce the psychological burden associated with these conditions, ultimately improving their quality of life. Similarly, corporate employees may use MBSR to manage work-related stress, while students might find it helpful in navigating academic pressures.

Moreover, the growing body of research on MBSR further validates its efficacy in stress and pain management. Studies have consistently shown that MBSR participants experience significant reductions in anxiety, depression, and perceived stress levels, alongside improvements in physical health markers. These findings provide compelling evidence supporting MBSR as a credible intervention for enhancing mental well-being and coping abilities.

In conclusion, MBSR stands as a testament to the power of mindfulness-based practices in contemporary healthcare. From its origins under Dr. Jon Kabat-Zinn's guidance to its global dissemination, MBSR has carved out a niche as a valuable tool for easing the burdens of stress and pain. Its capacity to complement traditional treatments while adapting to diverse populations has cemented its place as a leading approach in holistic health and wellness. Through continuous refinement and research, MBSR promises to remain an integral component of modern therapeutic strategies, offering hope and relief to those seeking alternative pathways to healing.

Core Principles of MBSR

Mindfulness-Based Stress Reduction (MBSR) serves as a beacon of hope for individuals grappling with the dual challenges of chronic pain and stress. At its core, MBSR pivots around foundational principles that invite participants to reimagine their relationship with pain and stress, transforming them from burdens into opportunities for growth and healing.

The essence of mindfulness is being present without judgment, a concept that seamlessly aligns with breaking the cycle of suffering. Often, when we're engulfed in pain or stress, our thoughts spiral into judgments—self-blame, despair, anger—that exacerbate our distress. Mindfulness offers an alternative: a gentle yet profound shift in focus towards the present moment. This mental discipline encourages individuals to observe their experiences without attaching labels or judgments. In doing so, they begin to see pain not as an enemy but as a part of their experience that warrants observation and understanding (Ackerman, 2019). By fostering this presence, mindfulness helps dissolve the cycles of negativity that often accompany chronic discomfort.

Complementing mindfulness is the cultivation of body awareness, an essential practice within MBSR that aids in tuning into physical sensations. Pain, by its nature, demands attention, but often this attention is framed in fear and resistance. Developing body awareness allows individuals to engage with their pain differently. Instead of resisting or fearing it, they can explore these sensations with curiosity. This exploration can illuminate how pain manifests and changes, providing insights that might otherwise remain hidden beneath layers of tension and anxiety (Hofmann & Gómez, 2018).

Furthermore, acceptance acts as an anchor in navigating life's storms with resilience. For many, resistance to pain or stressful situations compounds their difficulty; it's akin to fighting against a strong current. Acceptance involves embracing one's experiences as they are, without trying to alter or suppress them. This isn't a passive surrender but rather an active engagement with reality, acknowledging pain's presence while choosing how to respond. Through acceptance, individuals cultivate emotional resilience, gaining strength from facing challenges head-on rather than shying away from them (Ackerman, 2019).

A crucial element of the MBSR framework is practicing non-judgment, which invites participants to observe their thoughts and feelings impartially. This practice fosters a vital detachment from self-critical narratives, freeing individuals from the weight of constant self-evaluation. Non-judgment diminishes the internal pressure to categorize every experience as good or bad, right or wrong (Hofmann & Gómez, 2018). By letting go of this binary thinking, individuals may find relief from the stress and anxiety that frequently accompany chronic illness. They learn that their worth isn't tied to the absence of pain or negative emotions, but rather to their capacity to acknowledge and handle these states with grace.

Incorporating these foundational principles into daily life does more than mitigate pain; it transforms one's entire approach to living. Mindfulness and body awareness enhance the ability to stay grounded and attentive to the moment, leading to a greater appreciation of life despite its trials. As individuals embody acceptance and non-judgment, they discover a quiet strength that enables them to weather adversity with increased equanimity and fewer emotional upheavals.

The real power of MBSR lies in its accessibility and adaptability. It provides a structured yet flexible pathway toward healing, accommodating diverse needs and backgrounds. This versatility ensures that people who engage with MBSR aren't just handed a set of instructions—they're empowered to take an active role in their wellbeing journey. Whether through formal meditation practices or the subtle integration of mindfulness into everyday activities, participants have a range of tools at their disposal to support their ongoing efforts to manage stress and pain (Center for Mindfulness, 2017).

MBSR Techniques for Stress

Mindfulness-Based Stress Reduction (MBSR) offers a variety of techniques tailored to alleviate stress, foster relaxation, and manage chronic pain. At its heart, MBSR is about being present in the moment, an approach that can not only reduce anxiety but also improve one's overall quality of life. Let us delve into some of the key practices that form the core of MBSR.

One of the most fundamental techniques within MBSR is mindful meditation, which centers on focusing attention on the breath or bodily sensations. This practice has been shown to significantly lower stress levels and provides benefits that extend well beyond each session into daily life. By concentrating on the rhythm of your breathing, you learn to anchor your mind amidst the chaos, allowing stressors to drift away like clouds in the sky. The power of this simple act lies in its ability to cultivate a sense of calm and clarity, helping individuals to step back from their immediate reactions to stress. In practice, it's about finding a quiet space, sitting comfortably, and gently guiding your focus onto your breath. Whenever your mind begins to wander, as it naturally will, kindly redirect your attention back to the present moment. (Ackerman, 2019)

Complementing mindful meditation are body scan techniques. These involve a systematic focus on different parts of the body, aiding both relaxation and enhanced awareness of pain. During a body scan, the practitioner is guided through various regions of the body, noticing and acknowledging sensations without judgment. This method has particular value for those experiencing chronic pain, as it helps in identifying specific areas of tension or discomfort that might otherwise go unnoticed. The practice encourages a shift in perspective—from resisting or feeling overwhelmed by pain to observing it with curiosity and acceptance. Start by lying down or sitting comfortably, closing your eyes if you wish, and bringing attention to your toes, slowly moving upwards to your head, noting any sensations along the way. (Center for Mindfulness, 2017)

Another enriching practice in the MBSR repertoire is mindful walking. This technique brings mindfulness into everyday movement, transforming walking into a meditative experience that connects physical activity to mental clarity. It involves being fully present with each step—feeling the ground beneath your feet and noticing the subtle shifts in balance and motion. Such engagement fosters a deeper connection between mind and body, often resulting in a clearer mental state and reduced stress. To practice mindful walking, find a place where you can walk slowly without interruption. Start by standing still, taking deep breaths, and then begin walking at a leisurely pace, paying attention to each step and the sensations it brings. Whether indoors or outdoors, this exercise seamlessly integrates mindfulness into daily routines, making it accessible for most people. (Mindfulness-Based Stress Reduction (MBSR) - MBSR Exercises, n.d.)

While individual practices play a crucial role, the social aspect of MBSR cannot be overlooked. Group sessions offer invaluable support and shared experiences that foster a sense of community and accountability. These gatherings bring together individuals on similar journeys, creating a supportive network that enhances motivation and provides a platform for sharing insights and challenges. Being part of a group can amplify the benefits of MBSR, as participants learn from each other and celebrate collective progress. Moreover, the communal setting reinforces commitment to regular practice, an essential element for reaping long-term benefits. While guidelines aren't necessary for participation in these sessions, the emphasis remains on openness, listening, and nurturing a non-judgmental environment.

Research on MBSR Benefits

Mindfulness-Based Stress Reduction (MBSR) emerges as a compelling alternative to conventional stress and pain management techniques. With roots in meditation and yoga, clinical studies have explored its effectiveness in alleviating chronic pain and reducing stress over time. These studies consistently demonstrate significant improvements in various dimensions of well-being, underscoring the potential of MBSR to transform lives.

Clinical evidence highlights that MBSR participants often report decreased pain intensity and enhanced coping mechanisms. For instance, one study involving individuals with chronic back pain revealed that those who engaged in MBSR not only experienced reduced pain but also improved daily functioning compared to those receiving traditional care (Harris et al., 2023). Such findings emphasize how MBSR can mitigate physical discomfort while enhancing overall quality of life.

The profound impact of MBSR extends beyond numbers and statistics. Patient testimonials vividly illustrate how mindfulness practices have improved their real-world experiences. Many individuals have shared stories of awakening to new perspectives on their pain, finding solace in present-moment awareness, and discovering renewed hope amid struggles. For example, patients describe how mindfulness helps them accept discomfort without judgment, enabling them to respond to pain rather than react impulsively.

Compelling meta-analyses reinforce MBSR's efficacy across diverse populations. In a systematic review of randomized controlled trials, significant reductions in both pain and depressive symptoms were observed among participants practicing mindfulness meditation (Hilton et al., 2017). Notably, these analyses highlight consistent trends, suggesting that MBSR effectively fosters better mental health and enhances resilience against chronic pain's emotional toll.

Synthetic literature reviews reveal that MBSR offers distinct advantages over other stress reduction techniques. Comparatively, MBSR uniquely combines meditation and mindful movement, fostering holistic well-being. Its non-intrusive nature appeals to many seeking gentle yet potent interventions. Studies draw attention to the superior flexibility and adaptability of MBSR methods which can be tailored to individual preferences and needs, unlike more rigid traditional therapies.

However, it is worth noting some discrepancies in research outcomes. One study focusing on breast cancer survivors did not find significant benefits in managing neuropathic pain through group-based MBSR sessions (Harris et al., 2023). This variance underscores an important consideration: that the format and delivery of MBSR might impact its effectiveness, emphasizing the need for more personalized approaches.

Despite these occasional inconsistencies, a growing body of evidence supports MBSR's role in managing non-cancer pain, highlighting a crucial area for further exploration. However, access to high-quality MBSR programs remains limited in certain regions, posing challenges for those seeking alternatives to pharmacotherapy or invasive treatments. Addressing this gap involves expanding availability, exploring online formats, partnering with local community organizations, and utilizing easily accessible venues like pharmacies to provide greater opportunities for participation.

Among the barriers to accessing MBSR services are travel restrictions and limited awareness among potential beneficiaries. Surveys reveal that significant proportions of individuals are unfamiliar with MBSR or feel inadequately informed about its benefits (Harris et al., 2023). Raising awareness through education initiatives can help bridge this knowledge gap, empowering more individuals to explore mindfulness practice as a viable solution.

Beyond merely mitigating symptoms, MBSR fosters essential skills for long-term self-management of pain. The practice encourages mindfulness—a cornerstone of conscious living—enabling individuals to become attuned observers of their inner experiences. By cultivating awareness and nurturing non-reactive acceptance, practitioners can challenge limiting beliefs, build emotional resilience, and ultimately lead fuller and more fulfilling lives.

Patient narratives eloquently convey how MBSR transforms perspectives, allowing sufferers to view pain through a different lens. Living mindfully empowers these individuals to take charge of their circumstances, diminishing feelings of helplessness often associated with chronic pain conditions. Simple acts of focused breathing and intentional presence become invaluable allies against challenging sensations.

Implementing MBSR in Daily Life

Integrating Mindfulness-Based Stress Reduction (MBSR) into daily life can significantly enhance one's ability to manage stress and pain. This practice encourages a deeper connection with oneself, fostering mental clarity and emotional resilience. By following actionable steps, individuals can make mindfulness an intrinsic part of their routine, thus facilitating consistent self-care.

One effective way to incorporate MBSR into daily life is by scheduling dedicated moments for mindfulness practice. Allocating specific times each day allows you to establish a habit, promoting both commitment and consistency. Consider starting your day with mindfulness exercises such as mindful breathing or meditation. Such activities prepare your mind for the challenges ahead, providing a solid foundation upon which to build your daily experiences. Evening sessions can serve as a calming ritual, enabling you to unwind and reflect on the day's events. Consistency in these practices can gradually transform them into an essential component of your self-care regimen (Mental Health Foundation, 2022).

Creating a conducive mindfulness space is another impactful strategy. A designated area for engaging in mindfulness exercises enhances focus and tranquility. Whether it's a corner of your room or a spot in your garden, ensure that this space is free from distractions and imbued with elements that promote peace—such as soft lighting, calming scents, or cushions for comfort. The physical environment plays a critical role in anchoring your practice, allowing you to delve deeper into moments of reflection and serenity (Home, n.d.).

Mindfulness need not be confined to formal sessions; it can be smoothly integrated into routine tasks too. Everyday activities like walking, eating, or even washing dishes can become mindfulness opportunities. For example, during your morning walk, pay attention to the feeling of the ground beneath your feet and the rhythm of your breath. When eating, savor each bite, noting the textures and flavors, turning eating into a sensory experience. These practices help cultivate a state of awareness and presence in mundane tasks, transforming the ordinary into occasions for mindfulness exploration (Mental Health Foundation, 2022).

Community resources are invaluable for those looking to support and deepen their MBSR journey. Local groups often host mindfulness sessions, offering a sense of community and shared purpose. Engaging with others provides accountability, encouragement, and varied perspectives on mindfulness practice. Additionally, online platforms abound with resources, including guided meditations, forums, and courses tailored to different experience levels. These communities can offer the support needed to sustain motivation and navigate any obstacles encountered along the way (Home, n.d.).

Final Thoughts

In this chapter, we've explored the roots and evolution of Mindfulness-Based Stress Reduction (MBSR), discovering its role in helping individuals navigate the challenges of stress and pain through mindfulness practices. MBSR was pioneered by Dr. Jon Kabat-Zinn as a non-traditional therapeutic approach to complement conventional treatments. By promoting awareness and acceptance, it empowers people to engage with their experiences more mindfully, ultimately improving their ability to manage chronic conditions. From medical settings to global dissemination, MBSR's adaptability has allowed it to cater to diverse populations, providing relief and fostering resilience across various domains.

As we close this chapter, it's clear that MBSR's value lies not only in its efficacy but also in its accessibility and flexibility. These qualities make it an appealing option for those seeking manageable ways to enhance their well-being. The techniques outlined offer practical tools to integrate mindfulness into daily life, transforming how individuals relate to their pain. By embracing these methods, one can cultivate patience and self-awareness, opening pathways toward healing and a better quality of life. Through continued practice and community support, readers are encouraged to embark on their own journeys of discovery and healing, confident in the knowledge that they have a compassionate ally in MBSR.

Reference List

Ackerman, C. (2019, July 4). *MBSR: 25 Mindfulness-Based Stress Reduction Exercises and Courses.* PositivePsychology.com. https://positivepsychology.com/mindfulness-based-stress-reduction-mbsr/

Harris, K., Jackson, J. L., Webster, H. L., Farrow, J. A., Zhao, Y., & Hohmann, L. (2023, September 21). *Mindfulness-Based Stress Reduction (MBSR) for Chronic Pain Management in the Community Pharmacy Setting: A Cross-*

Sectional Survey of the General Public's Knowledge and Perceptions. Pharmacy; Multidisciplinary Digital Publishing Institute. https://doi.org/10.3390/pharmacy11050150

Home. (n.d.). Mindfulness Based Stress Reduction. https://mbsrtraining.com/

Hofmann, S. G., & Gómez, A. F. (2018). *Mindfulness-Based Interventions for Anxiety and Depression*. Psychiatric Clinics of North America. https://doi.org/10.1016/j.psc.2017.08.008

Hilton, L., Hempel, S., Ewing, B. A., Apaydin, E., Xenakis, L., Newberry, S., Colaiaco, B., Maher, A. R., Shanman, R. M., Sorbero, M. E., & Maglione, M. A. (2017, September 22). *Mindfulness meditation for chronic pain: Systematic review and meta-analysis*. Annals of Behavioral Medicine. https://doi.org/10.1007/s12160-016-9844-2

History of MBSR. (n.d.). MBSR Collaborative. https://mbsrcollaborative.com/history-of-mbsr

Mindfulness-based stress reduction (MBSR) - MBSR exercises. (n.d.). Guy's and St Thomas' NHS Foundation Trust. https://www.guysandstthomas.nhs.uk/health-information/mindfulness-based-stress-reduction-mbsr/mbsr-exercises

Mental Health Foundation. (2022). *How to look after your mental health using mindfulness*. Www.mentalhealth.org.uk. https://www.mentalhealth.org.uk/explore-mental-health/publications/how-look-after-your-mental-health-using-mindfulness

Niazi, A. K., & Niazi, S. K. (2011). *Mindfulness-based Stress reduction: a non-pharmacological Approach for Chronic*

Illnesses. North American Journal of Medical Sciences. https://doi.org/10.4297/najms.2011.320

CHAPTER 8

Adapting Mindfulness to Different Pain Conditions

Adapting mindfulness to different pain conditions offers a promising pathway to manage discomfort and improve quality of life. Pain, often an unwelcome companion, disrupts daily routines, affects emotional balance, and clouds mental clarity. Despite the inevitable presence of pain in life, understanding that it does not have to dominate our existence is vital. Mindfulness, with its roots in awareness and acceptance, provides individuals with the tools to approach pain with a clear, compassionate mind. This chapter is dedicated to exploring how these practices can be tailored for varying conditions, offering hope and tangible strategies for those seeking relief. Whether it's back pain, arthritis, fibromyalgia, or even tension headaches, the journey toward managing pain begins by cultivating a deeper connection between body and mind.

Throughout this chapter, we delve into specific strategies that align with particular pain conditions, exploring how simple adjustments to mindfulness techniques can lead to profound changes. You will discover how mindful posture awareness plays a crucial role in alleviating chronic back pain, allowing for healthier movement and reduced physical tension. For arthritis sufferers, gentle movement becomes a dance of balance, promoting joint flexibility while fostering harmony between body and soul. Those managing fibromyalgia will find comfort in pacing techniques that honor the body's limitations without judgment, ensuring energy reserves are wisely spent. Moreover, for tension headache sufferers, identifying personal triggers and practicing relaxation techniques can become powerful allies. Each discussion highlights the benefits of personalized mindfulness approaches, demonstrating that with patience and practice, one can transform their relationship with pain. As you venture through these insights, may you find inspiration and encouragement to embrace mindfulness as a valuable ally in your journey towards well-being.

Chronic Back Pain

Managing chronic back pain through mindfulness involves a thoughtful, multifaceted approach that addresses physical alignment, movement, emotional acceptance, and relaxation techniques. Let's dive into each aspect to better understand how these strategies can alleviate discomfort.

Mindful Posture Awareness

Posture plays a crucial role in managing back pain. By bringing mindful awareness to your posture, you can significantly reduce spine pressure and alleviate discomfort. This awareness involves tuning into your body's natural alignment, ensuring that your head, shoulders, and pelvis are in line, thus reducing strain on the back muscles. Start by observing your posture during everyday activities like sitting, standing, or working at a desk. Notice any habitual slouching or tension. Use this awareness to gently correct your posture by imagining a string pulling from the top of your head, aligning your spine. Over time, mindful posture awareness can become an automatic habit, contributing to ongoing pain relief. Consistent practice of mindful posture not only alleviates immediate discomfort but also fosters long-term spinal health and prevents future back issues (<i>Mindfulness Techniques for Pain Management</i>, n.d.).

Gentle Movement Practices

Incorporating gentle movement practices is another effective mindfulness strategy. Techniques such as yoga or tai chi can enhance circulation and improve respiratory function, contributing to overall physical well-being. These movements should be slow, intentional, and focused. As you move, pay close attention to how your muscles and joints feel, noting any areas of tightness without forcing or rushing movements. Breathing deeply during these exercises further aids in relaxing tense areas and improving oxygen flow throughout the body. Studies have shown that patients with chronic low back pain experience significant reductions in pain when engaging in mindful exercises compared to traditional strength or stretching workouts (<i>Mindfulness Techniques for Pain Management</i>, n.d.). The rhythmic and mindful nature of these practices helps create a sense of harmony between the mind and body, ultimately reducing pain perception and enhancing quality of life (Dubey & Muley, 2023).

Pain Acceptance Strategies

Accepting pain without judgment can lead to reduced emotional distress and stress. It's important to acknowledge that pain is a part of your current experience without labeling it as good or bad. This doesn't mean resigning to pain but recognizing it without allowing it to dominate your emotions. One effective technique involves using breath as an anchor; inhale deeply, acknowledging the presence of pain, and exhale while releasing any tension or judgment related to it. Embracing this non-judgmental awareness can decrease the grip of negative emotions often associated with chronic pain, thereby reducing its psychological impact (*Mindfulness Techniques for Pain Management*, n.d.). Recognizing and accepting pain removes the additional burden of emotional suffering and empowers individuals to focus their energy on proactive coping mechanisms.

Visualization Techniques

Finally, visualization techniques provide a mental space for relaxation and healing. By creating calming visual images in your mind, you can induce relaxation, distract from pain, and promote healing. Visualization can involve imagining a warm, soothing light enveloping areas of discomfort or picturing yourself in a peaceful setting like a sunny beach or serene forest. As these mental images bring about a state of calmness, they help release tension and alter one's perception of pain. This technique is rooted in the principle that the mind can influence bodily sensations, offering a pathway to reduce stress and foster an environment conducive to healing. Visualization not only encourages relaxation but also enhances one's capacity to cope with pain more effectively (Dubey & Muley, 2023).

Arthritis and Joint Pain

Adapting mindfulness techniques to manage arthritis and joint pain can offer powerful ways to navigate the challenges imposed by these conditions. By tailoring specific practices, individuals can find pathways to not only manage pain but also improve their overall quality of life.

Mindful movement stands out as a significant practice for those dealing with arthritis. Integrating exercises like yoga or tai chi can be particularly beneficial. These forms of mindful movement focus on gentle, deliberate motions that improve joint flexibility while fostering a deep connection between mind and body (Sani et al., 2023). Yoga, with its varied poses and stretches, encourages smoother joint movement without overexertion, making it ideal for arthritis sufferers. Similarly, tai chi combines slow, flowing movements with precise breathing techniques, promoting balance and relaxation. This kind of exercise boosts physical health and supports mental well-being, acting as a natural antidote to stress and depression associated with chronic pain (The, 2023).

Expanding on these benefits, conducting body scans focused specifically on the joints is another fruitful mindfulness approach. This involves lying down in a comfortable position and mentally scanning your body, with particular attention to areas of discomfort or tension. Bringing awareness to painful areas allows you to observe sensations without judgment, fostering self-awareness and acceptance. Through this practice, one can learn to embrace limitations with compassion rather than resistance (The, 2023). Consistent body scans can improve emotional resilience, enabling individuals to develop proactive coping strategies in the face of ongoing pain.

Beyond physical practices, applying mindfulness techniques to calm inflammation can also make a substantial difference. Mindfulness reduces stress hormones like cortisol, which can exacerbate inflammation in the body. Engaging in simple practices such as mindful breathing helps in calming the nervous system, which may lead to a reduction in pain perception (The, 2023). Taking even a few minutes each day to focus solely on the breath—breathing in slowly through the nose and exhaling through the mouth—can create a profound sense of peace and reduce the impact of inflammatory signals.

Building emotional resilience is crucial when living with the persistent challenge of arthritis. While physical pain is often the most immediate concern, the emotional toll should not be underestimated. Developing resilience through mindfulness provides tools for better emotional regulation and stress management. By acknowledging the presence of pain and accepting it without judgment, individuals can cultivate a more compassionate relationship with their bodies. Emotional resilience is further strengthened by practicing gratitude and focusing on positive aspects of life despite the difficulties posed by chronic pain (The, 2023). This mindset shift can significantly reduce anxiety and depression, common co-travelers with arthritis.

Moreover, mindfulness fosters an environment where proactive coping strategies can thrive. Recognizing that pain is indeed a part of life but does not need to control it opens up possibilities for enriched experiences. Embracing these principles, people can engage in activities they love, restoring joy and purpose. Sharing these insights with others, perhaps through support groups or mindfulness classes, can create a community of shared understanding and encouragement (Sani et al., 2023). Knowing you're not alone in your journey can be incredibly empowering, providing additional motivation to adhere to mindfulness practices consistently.

Incorporating mindfulness into daily routine requires dedication and patience. Like any skill, mindfulness develops gradually and builds over time. Encouragement to begin with small, manageable sessions can ease any overwhelming feelings about committing to a new practice. Over time, increasing the duration and integrating different techniques— mindful breathing, movement, and meditation—can provide comprehensive relief from both physical and emotional symptoms associated with arthritis (The, 2023).

For those new to mindfulness, seeking guidance can be beneficial. Joining a class or working with a coach offers personalized instructions and structured growth. Moreover, using digital resources like mindfulness apps facilitates convenient access to guided practices. These platforms can be instrumental in maintaining consistency and providing motivation, extending the reach of mindfulness beyond traditional settings (The, 2023).

Fibromyalgia Management

Fibromyalgia, a chronic condition characterized by widespread pain and profound fatigue, often necessitates an adaptable approach for effective management. One promising avenue is the integration of mindfulness practices tailored to address the unique challenges presented by fibromyalgia symptoms. These practices not only help in managing physical discomfort but also contribute significantly to emotional and mental well-being, thereby enhancing overall quality of life.

Pacing techniques stand out as a crucial component in mindfulness practice for individuals with fibromyalgia. The concept of pacing involves the careful balancing of activity and rest, which can be pivotal in preventing the exacerbation of symptoms. For instance, a person might break down tasks into smaller, manageable units interspersed with periods of rest, rather than attempting to complete activities in one go. This mindful distribution of energy helps prevent overexertion and the subsequent cycle of increased pain and fatigue commonly experienced by those with fibromyalgia. By remaining attuned to their body's signals, individuals can learn to anticipate and respond to fatigue before it leads to a flare-up, making daily living more manageable (<i>5 Mindfulness Techniques to Help Cope with Chronic Pain</i>, 2024).

Grounding exercises are another valuable mindfulness tool for fibromyalgia sufferers. These exercises aim to shift attention away from pain and promote emotional stability. Grounding might involve simple practices such as focusing on deep breathing, connecting with nature through a gentle walk, or employing sensory awareness exercises that anchor the individual in the present moment. By redirecting focus to immediate sensory inputs—the feel of the ground underfoot, the sound of rustling leaves—individuals can cultivate a sense of calmness and diminish the overwhelming focus on pain. Such practices support emotional well-being by encouraging positivity and reducing stress and anxiety, common companions of chronic pain conditions (<i>Mindfulness for Fibromyalgia</i>, 2022).

Managing fatigue effectively through mindfulness is integral for those battling fibromyalgia. Fatigue is often more debilitating than the pain itself, and learning to manage it can greatly improve one's quality of life. Mindfulness encourages the development of personalized strategies to cope with this persistent fatigue. Techniques may include conscious energy allocation, where individuals set priorities and allocate their limited energy reserves wisely. It could also involve the use of restorative yoga or meditation sessions aimed specifically at replenishing energy levels. These mindfulness-based interventions not only help in conserving energy but also empower individuals to take an active role in their health management (<i>Mindfulness for Fibromyalgia</i>, 2022).

While self-compassion may not directly alleviate fibromyalgia symptoms, nurturing a compassionate mindset forms a fundamental aspect of mindfulness practice. Cultivating self-compassion entails recognizing one's struggles without judgment and offering oneself kindness and understanding. This nurtures resilience, reduces self-criticism, and fosters a supportive inner dialogue that is particularly beneficial during moments of heightened discomfort or emotional distress. By being gentle with themselves, individuals can better navigate the daily challenges posed by fibromyalgia, thus promoting a more balanced and peaceful state of mind. As research indicates, letting go of attachment to painful experiences can enhance the effectiveness of mindfulness, helping individuals transform their relationship with pain from adversarial to accepting (<i>5 Mindfulness Techniques to Help Cope with Chronic Pain</i>, 2024).

Irritable Bowel Syndrome

Mindfulness has emerged as a powerful tool for managing various health conditions, including Irritable Bowel Syndrome (IBS). By focusing on mindfulness strategies, individuals suffering from IBS can gain relief from their symptoms and improve their quality of life. One central aspect of integrating mindfulness into daily life is the practice of mindful eating. This involves paying close attention to each bite of food, experiencing the flavors and textures without judgment, and being aware of how different foods impact the digestive system. Through mindful eating, individuals can better understand which foods act as triggers for their IBS symptoms, thereby improving digestion and reducing discomfort.

Developing body awareness is another key strategy in managing IBS through mindfulness. When individuals become more attuned to the sensations in their bodies, they can differentiate between emotional and physical discomfort, which is crucial for those with IBS who often experience stress-related symptoms. This heightened awareness allows them to identify when emotions are impacting their gut health and take proactive steps to address these emotions before they exacerbate physical symptoms. Body scans and other mindfulness exercises can help cultivate this awareness, leading to improved management of IBS symptoms.

Diaphragmatic breathing techniques offer a practical method for alleviating anxiety and digestive discomfort associated with IBS. By engaging in deep, controlled breathing, individuals can activate their parasympathetic nervous system, promoting relaxation and reducing stress-induced digestive issues. Practicing diaphragmatic breathing regularly can result in lower anxiety levels and mitigate the severity of IBS symptoms, offering a natural way to manage this often debilitating condition.

Stress reduction strategies are integral to using mindfulness for IBS management, as stress is a well-known contributor to gastrointestinal issues. Techniques such as meditation, progressive muscle relaxation, and guided imagery can help individuals decrease their overall stress levels, thereby minimizing the impact of stress on their digestive health. Engaging in these practices consistently not only reduces anxiety but also supports long-term gastrointestinal health by fostering a calmer, more balanced state of mind.

The connection between the brain and gut plays a significant role in how IBS symptoms manifest. The brain-gut axis involves continuous communication between these two entities, meaning that emotional and cognitive states can directly influence gut function. By implementing mindfulness practices, individuals can alter their perception of gut sensations and decrease maladaptive cognitions that contribute to symptom flare-ups. Psychological therapies, as highlighted in the Evidence-Based Position Statement on the Management of Irritable Bowel Syndrome, are effective in relieving IBS symptoms due to their ability to modulate the brain-gut interaction (Gaylord et al., 2011).

Moreover, mindfulness-based stress reduction (MBSR) programs have demonstrated efficacy in treating various chronic health conditions, including gastrointestinal disorders (Cherpak, 2019). These programs incorporate practices like diaphragmatic breathing and body scans, effectively targeting IBS symptoms by addressing both physiological and psychological components. The evidence supporting MBSR for IBS underscores the significance of mindfulness in managing this condition.

Studies have shown that mindfulness can induce changes in neural circuits related to interoception and emotion regulation, which are vital for managing IBS (Gaylord et al., 2011). By enhancing attentional control and reducing distress caused by heightened pain perception, mindfulness training offers a therapeutic approach tailored to the unique challenges faced by individuals with IBS.

Mindful eating transforms the act of eating into an opportunity for reflection and self-discovery. By shifting focus to the sensory experience of eating, individuals can break free from habitual, unconscious eating patterns that may exacerbate IBS symptoms. This practice encourages exploration of the complex relationship between thoughts, feelings, and physiological responses, ultimately fostering healthier eating habits and improved digestive function (Cherpak, 2019).

Building resilience to stress through mindfulness also facilitates better management of IBS. Stress disrupts digestive function, causing variations in motility and exacerbating symptoms such as pain and bloating. Mindfulness practices strengthen an individual's ability to cope with stress, promoting a stable internal environment that supports digestive health.

Tension Headaches

Incorporating mindfulness practices into daily routines can be a transformative approach for those struggling with tension headaches. These headaches, often linked to stress and muscle tension, can significantly disrupt daily activities and overall well-being. By tailoring mindfulness techniques specifically for this condition, individuals can find relief and improve their quality of life.

Relaxation techniques like guided imagery and progressive muscle relaxation are effective tools in alleviating the physical and mental tension that accompanies headaches. Guided imagery involves visualizing calming scenes or experiences, allowing the mind to escape from stressors and reduce the perception of pain. This visualization can be led by oneself or through audio guides that prompt the mind to wander to peaceful environments. Progressive muscle relaxation, on the other hand, is a systematic process of tensing and then relaxing different muscle groups. It helps in identifying where stress is primarily stored and gradually easing the tension throughout the body. Studies have shown that these techniques not only help in reducing headache intensity but also promote a sense of overall relaxation (Mayo Clinic, 2023).

Identifying habitual triggers is another crucial step in managing tension headaches. Often, lifestyle factors such as irregular meal times, poor sleep patterns, and certain foods or environmental stimuli contribute to the onset of headaches. Keeping a headache diary can be instrumental in recognizing patterns and triggers. Documenting occurrences of headaches alongside potential triggers—such as specific foods, strenuous activities, or emotional stress—empowers individuals to make informed lifestyle changes. For instance, if a particular food triggers a headache, avoiding it in the future can prevent distress. Over time, this proactive management aids in reducing the frequency and severity of tension headaches (tylorBennett, 2024).

Another important factor to consider is posture awareness. In today's digital age, many people spend significant hours sitting at desks or using electronic devices, often leading to poor posture. Tension builds up in the neck and shoulders, which can exacerbate headaches. Practicing good posture—sitting with a straight back, shoulders relaxed, and feet flat on the floor—can prevent unnecessary strain. Ergonomic adjustments, such as using supportive chairs and adjusting screen heights, further enhance comfort. Regularly checking one's posture and making necessary corrections becomes a mindful activity that helps in mitigating tension build-up over time (tylorBennett, 2024).

Meditation plays a pivotal role in maintaining mental relaxation and minimizing headache intensity. Various studies highlight meditation's effectiveness in managing chronic pain conditions, including tension headaches. Mindfulness meditation, in particular, focuses on breathing and awareness of the present moment. By concentrating on slow, deep breaths and calmly acknowledging thoughts without judgment, one can create a mental state conducive to relaxation. This practice helps diminish the stress response, thereby lessening the headache's impact. Additionally, other forms of meditation like yoga and tai chi, which incorporate gentle movements with breath control, offer both physical relaxation and enhanced mental clarity (Mayo Clinic, 2023).

Implementing these mindfulness practices requires consistency and patience. It's essential for individuals to experiment with different techniques to discover what suits them best. Whether it's starting the day with a brief meditation session, engaging in guided imagery before sleep, or taking regular breaks to evaluate posture, each small step contributes to long-term headache management. Ultimately, integrating these practices fosters a mindful living approach, emphasizing awareness and proactive care in daily routines.

Summary and Reflections

Throughout this chapter, we've explored how mindfulness can be tailored to address the unique challenges of managing pain from various chronic conditions. Whether it's tuning into your posture to ease back strain, gracefully moving through yoga poses to soothe arthritis, or practicing grounding exercises for fibromyalgia, these mindful practices are designed to nurture both body and mind. The goal is to empower you with techniques that not only relieve physical discomfort but also enhance emotional resilience. Each small step toward integrating mindfulness invites a deeper understanding of your body's needs and encourages compassionate self-care.

As you reflect on these strategies, remember that the journey to wellness is deeply personal. Embracing mindfulness as part of your daily routine requires patience and kindness toward yourself. It's about finding balance in every breath, accepting setbacks with grace, and celebrating progress. By weaving these practices into your life, you open the door to improved well-being and a more meaningful relationship with your body. May these insights serve as a gentle guide, leading you along a path of healing and hope.

Reference List

5 Mindfulness Techniques to Help Cope With Chronic Pain. (2024). Psychology Today. https://www.psychologytoday.com/intl/blog/contemplative-psychology/202402/5-mindfulness-techniques-to-help-cope-with-chronic-pain

Cherpak, C. E. (2019, August). *Mindful Eating: A Review Of How The Stress-Digestion-Mindfulness Triad May Modulate And Improve Gastrointestinal And Digestive Function.* Integrative Medicine: A Clinician's Journal. https://pmc.ncbi.nlm.nih.gov/articles/PMC7219460/

Dubey, A., & Muley, P. A. (2023, November 22). *Meditation: A Promising Approach for Alleviating Chronic Pain.* Cureus. https://doi.org/10.7759/cureus.49244

Gaylord, S. A., Palsson, O. S., Garland, E. L., Faurot, K. R., Coble, R. S., Mann, D. J., Frey, W., Leniek, K., & Whitehead, W. E. (2011, September). *Mindfulness Training Reduces the Severity of Irritable Bowel Syndrome in Women: Results of a Randomized Controlled Trial.* American Journal of Gastroenterology. https://doi.org/10.1038/ajg.2011.184

Mindfulness Techniques For Pain Management. (n.d.). Physiopedia. https://www.physio-pedia.com/Mindfulness_Techniques_For_Pain_Management

Mayo Clinic. (2023, December 14). *Meditation: A simple, fast way to reduce stress.* Mayo Clinic. https://www.mayoclinic.org/tests-procedures/meditation/in-depth/meditation/art-20045858

Mindfulness for Fibromyalgia. (2022, May 13). Breathworks. https://www.breathworks-mindfulness.org.uk/blog/mindfulness-for-fibromyalgia

Sani, N. A., Yusoff, S. S. M., Norhayati, M. N., & Zainudin, A. M. (2023, February 5). *Tai Chi Exercise for Mental and Physical Well-Being in Patients with Depressive Symptoms: A Systematic Review and Meta-Analysis.* International Journal of Environmental Research and Public Health. https://doi.org/10.3390/ijerph20042828

The. (2023). *The Power of Mindfulness: Easing Arthritis Pain and Improving Well Being.* Arthritis Queensland. https://www.arthritis.org.au/arthritis/arthritis-insights/positive-health-habits/the-power-of-mindfulness-easing-arthritis-pain-and-improving-well-being/

tylorBennett. (2024, September 24). *Pain Management for Tension Headaches - Eastside Ideal Health Redmond.* Eastside Ideal Health Redmond. https://www.eastsideidealhealth.com/pain-management-for-tension-headaches/

CHAPTER 9

Integrating Mindfulness with Medical Treatments

Integrating mindfulness with medical treatments opens a doorway to a more profound understanding of pain management. This chapter explores the harmonious blend of traditional medical practices and mindfulness techniques, offering readers innovative ways to address chronic pain conditions. In modern healthcare, the fusion of these approaches can provide individuals with unique strategies that not only target physical symptoms but also nurture emotional and mental well-being. By tapping into the power of mindfulness, patients are equipped to navigate their pain with greater awareness and resilience. Although mindfulness might seem unconventional in a medical context, its integration has the potential to transform how individuals perceive and interact with their discomfort, leading to improved overall health outcomes.

The chapter unfolds by delving into the collaborative efforts needed between healthcare providers and patients to incorporate mindfulness into treatment plans effectively. Readers will journey through topics such as communication, patient empowerment, and the pivotal role of customized care strategies that resonate personally with each individual. It highlights the importance of education for both patients and providers, ensuring they are well-versed in mindfulness techniques and their benefits. Discussions include how coordinated care enhances treatment efficacy and prevents conflicts, while personalized mindfulness interventions elevate patient engagement and adherence. The exploration extends to interprofessional cooperation within healthcare, emphasizing the need for unified perspectives in crafting holistic treatment plans. Ultimately, this chapter invites readers to reimagine chronic pain management, where mindfulness and medical treatments work hand-in-hand to create a supportive, patient-centered environment dedicated to healing and growth.

Collaboration with Healthcare Providers

Enhancing treatment outcomes through collaborative healthcare efforts involves engaging patients as active participants in their health journey. Establishing open communication channels between patients and healthcare providers is crucial. This fosters a holistic approach where each voice is valued, leading to more personalized care. When patients communicate openly with their providers, they can express concerns, preferences, and goals more clearly. This ensures that their unique needs are considered in treatment planning, creating a sense of partnership rather than a one-sided directive.

Involving patients in decision-making not only boosts satisfaction but also improves adherence to treatment plans. By empowering individuals to be part of the decisions affecting their health, they are more likely to commit to recommended practices. When patients understand why certain treatments are chosen, and how these choices align with their personal goals, they become motivated allies in their healing process. According to research from the Wildflower Center for Emotional Health, effective care coordination significantly enhances patient outcomes by ensuring their involvement in setting health goals (CST (she/her), 2023).

Coordinated care plays a vital role in maintaining consistency and reducing the likelihood of conflicting treatments. In a complex healthcare system, where multiple specialists might be involved, seamless coordination is essential to avoid misunderstandings or duplications. Effective communication among all members of the healthcare team helps ensure that treatments are harmonized and informed by the same goals. For instance, coordinating medications and therapeutic interventions can prevent adverse interactions, thereby maximizing the effectiveness of the overall treatment strategy. Rosen's work underscores the significance of structured teamwork in healthcare, advocating for evidence-based coordination to improve patient safety and quality of care (Rosen, 2019).

Educating healthcare providers on mindfulness techniques further strengthens the integration of mindfulness into medical treatments. When providers are confident in recommending these practices, it empowers them to offer a broader spectrum of therapeutic options that complement traditional methods. Training sessions that introduce the principles and benefits of mindfulness enhance providers' ability to suggest appropriate exercises tailored to each patient's needs. This not only expands their skill set but also enriches the provider-patient relationship by opening up new avenues for dialogue about holistic care strategies.

Building a partnership between patients and providers requires transparency and trust. Guiding both parties in understanding the importance of mutual respect and shared objectives is key to this process. Providers should emphasize the value of listening and responding to patient feedback as a means of fostering trust. When patients feel heard and understood, they are more likely to engage actively in their treatment plans and collaborate enthusiastically on setting achievable health targets.

Effective communication is foundational yet often overlooked in clinical settings. It's important for healthcare professionals to practice clear communication styles that are accessible and engaging for patients from diverse backgrounds. Techniques such as active listening and using layman's terms can bridge potential gaps, making complex medical information comprehensible. Training programs focused on communication skills can help providers refine their approaches, thereby facilitating better patient-provider interactions. Research highlights the critical nature of communication in preventing errors and improving overall care delivery, as emphasized by experts studying teamwork dynamics in healthcare (Rosen, 2019).

Collaborative approaches extend beyond the patient-provider relationship to include interprofessional cooperation within the healthcare system. By sharing insights, experiences, and updates across disciplines, a more comprehensive picture of a patient's health can be developed. Interdisciplinary meetings and case discussions provide opportunities for different specialties to align their perspectives and formulate cohesive treatment plans. Such collaborations are particularly beneficial for managing chronic conditions where multifaceted care approaches are required to address the wide range of symptoms and impacts.

Patients empowered by knowledge become advocates for their health, asking questions, seeking alternatives, and making choices aligned with their values and circumstances. Educational resources provided during consultations equip patients with the tools needed to make informed decisions. Offering materials that explain the rationale behind treatment options and potential outcomes encourages patients to take ownership of their health journeys. According to studies, patient activation, which refers to the level at which individuals understand their health condition and manage their care, correlates positively with improved health outcomes and cost efficiencies (CST (she/her), 2023).

Mindfulness in Physical Therapy

Integrating mindfulness into physical therapy can significantly boost patient engagement and enhance the therapeutic process. This approach centers around using mindfulness to foster a deeper connection between the mind and body, thereby improving the efficacy of physical therapy. By enhancing body awareness through mindful movement, patients become more attuned to their bodies, which allows them to participate actively in their rehabilitation. Mindful movement involves paying attention to each sensation and motion during exercise, helping patients understand their physical responses and limitations better.

Patients managing chronic pain often find themselves disconnected from their bodies due to discomfort. However, incorporating mindfulness-based exercises helps individuals remain grounded and present during therapy sessions. These exercises encourage patients to observe their sensations without judgment, empowering them to manage discomfort more effectively. For instance, by focusing on their breathing, patients can redirect their attention away from pain, creating a calmer state that makes it easier to engage with physical activities.

Therapist training is fundamental to successfully integrating mindfulness into physical therapy. When therapists are equipped with skills to tailor mindfulness strategies, they can address the unique needs of each patient. Training programs can focus on teaching therapists how to incorporate mindfulness techniques seamlessly into traditional therapy frameworks. For example, therapists might use guided meditation or visualization exercises to complement physical routines, ensuring these interventions are accessible and relevant to the patient's condition.

Monitoring progress with mindfulness offers valuable insights into the rehabilitation process. Patients who practice mindfulness often report improved mental clarity and emotional resilience, factors that contribute to better rehabilitation outcomes. Through mindfulness assessments, therapists can track subtle changes in a patient's recovery journey that might otherwise go unnoticed. This nuanced understanding enables therapists to adjust treatment plans proactively, maximizing their effectiveness.

The integration of mindfulness in physical therapy doesn't just benefit the patient's physical health; it also enhances their overall well-being. Studies have shown that mindfulness practices can reduce stress and improve mood, leading to a more holistic recovery experience (Hardison & Roll, 2016). Moreover, as patients become more engaged, they are likely to adhere better to their therapy regimens, further accelerating their recovery.

The potential for mindfulness to transform physical therapy is supported by research indicating its efficacy in various medical contexts. While existing studies provide promising evidence, there is room for further exploration to refine these approaches for different settings and populations (Watson et al.,

2022). This ongoing research is crucial to understanding best practices and ensuring mindfulness strategies are implemented effectively across diverse healthcare environments.

Incorporating shared decision-making into this mindfulness-centered approach can empower patients further. By involving patients in their treatment planning, therapists can foster a sense of ownership over the recovery process, encouraging active participation. Patients who feel heard and valued are more likely to engage with their therapy meaningfully, enhancing the likelihood of successful outcomes.

Ultimately, the fusion of mindfulness and physical therapy has the potential to revolutionize patient care. As therapists gain a deeper understanding of mindfulness techniques and patients embrace these practices, the therapeutic relationship becomes more collaborative and impactful. This integration not only addresses the physical aspects of rehabilitation but also considers the emotional and psychological dimensions, fostering a comprehensive healing environment.

Complementary Alternative Medicine

Incorporating mindfulness practices with complementary and alternative medicine (CAM) techniques can provide a well-rounded, effective approach to pain management. Mindfulness, defined as the practice of being present and fully engaged in the current moment without judgment or distraction, has shown significant potential in enhancing the efficacy of various therapies such as acupuncture and massage. The American College of Physicians suggests nonpharmacologic approaches, including mindfulness-based stress reduction and acupuncture, for managing chronic low-back pain—a testament to the growing recognition of these integrative methods (<i>Chronic Pain and Complementary Health Approaches: Usefulness and Safety</i>, 2023).

Research indicates that when combined with CAM, mindfulness practices can help amplify therapeutic effects. For instance, acupuncture, which relies on balancing energy flow within the body, can be enhanced by the focused attention cultivated through mindfulness. Patients adopting both practices report heightened relaxation and a greater sense of bodily awareness, which may contribute to more profound healing experiences (Tabish, 2008). Similarly, massage therapy, known for its benefits in reducing muscle tension and improving circulation, can achieve even deeper results when clients engage in mindful breathing and awareness during sessions. This synergy between mindfulness and traditional techniques highlights the inherent adaptability of integrative health strategies.

Case studies serve as compelling narratives that illustrate the successful integration of mindfulness with CAM. Take, for example, a patient struggling with fibromyalgia, who found significant relief through a tailored regimen combining tai chi and mindful meditation. Over several months, this individual reported reduced pain levels and improved mobility, underscoring mindfulness's role in enhancing tai chi's therapeutic outcomes. Such examples not only affirm the benefits of this holistic approach but also encourage others to explore similar paths toward wellness. Publishing and sharing these stories create a ripple effect, inspiring healthcare providers and patients alike to consider comprehensive pain management plans that embrace both CAM and mindfulness.

Ensuring safety when integrating mindfulness and CAM is paramount. Open discussions about alternative methods between patients and healthcare providers establish a foundation of trust. It's crucial for practitioners to communicate clearly about what each therapy entails, its potential benefits and limitations, and any associated risks. This open communication helps patients make informed decisions about their treatment options and fosters an environment where they feel comfortable expressing concerns and preferences. Moreover, transparency about the evidence supporting these practices reassures patients about their safety and effectiveness, making them more likely to adhere to and benefit from their treatment plans.

A patient-centric approach, emphasizing personalized care, is essential when integrating mindfulness with CAM. Each individual's experience with pain is unique, demanding treatment plans tailored to personal needs and preferences. By prioritizing patient involvement in selecting therapies that resonate with them personally, healthcare providers can ensure higher degrees of engagement and satisfaction. Acknowledging cultural and spiritual beliefs, lifestyle factors, and emotional readiness for certain interventions empowers patients, making them active participants in their healing journey.

Moreover, incorporating mindfulness offers the opportunity to align treatment approaches with individual goals and preferences. For those with chronic pain, maintaining agency over their health choices enhances psychological well-being, promoting resilience and a positive outlook on recovery. Recognizing and valuing the distinct perspectives each patient brings allows for more nuanced and effective care, creating a partnership rooted in mutual respect and understanding.

While the integration of mindfulness and CAM presents promising pathways to improved health outcomes, it is important to recognize the need for continued research and education in this field. Educating patients and healthcare professionals about the potentials and limitations of these combined therapies ensures informed decision-making and broadens acceptance within conventional medical settings. As emerging evidence continues to support mindfulness and CAM's synergistic benefits, fostering ongoing dialogue and research will drive innovation in pain management strategies, ultimately improving the quality of life for many individuals.

Patient-Centered Care

In chronic pain management, integrating mindfulness with medical treatments offers a transformative path towards fostering collaboration and respect between healthcare providers and patients. This holistic approach emphasizes the importance of understanding each patient's unique needs and harnessing their input to create more effective treatment plans.

Personalizing mindfulness interventions is vital as it significantly enhances patient engagement. Each individual experiences chronic pain differently, influenced by various physical, emotional, and environmental factors. Mindfulness practices can be tailored to address these personal nuances, whether through specific meditation techniques, relaxation exercises, or mindful movement strategies. For instance, one patient might find relief in guided imagery, while another benefits more from breath-focused meditation. Personalization aligns therapeutic interventions with individual preferences, increasing the likelihood of active participation and sustained practice. As individualized care grows, so does the patient's commitment to their health journey, cultivating a deeper sense of agency over their condition (Themelis & Tang, 2023).

Encouraging patients to articulate their needs and experiences proves pivotal in enhancing psychological well-being. Open dialogue invites patients to communicate their perceptions of pain and its impacts on their lives, helping healthcare providers understand not just the physical symptoms but also the mental and emotional burdens accompanying chronic pain. When patients feel heard, they gain confidence in their role within the treatment process, which can lead to improved relationships with caregivers. This collaborative environment enables practitioners to craft therapy plans that are empathetic and responsive to genuine patient concerns, further strengthening therapeutic alliances.

Holistic assessments, supported by mindfulness, offer a comprehensive approach to recognizing mental health factors often intertwined with chronic pain. Chronic pain can lead to anxiety, depression, and other mental health challenges that exacerbate physical symptoms. Mindfulness-based evaluation tools help in identifying these co-occurring issues, allowing for the development of integrated treatment models that cater to both mind and body. Practicing mindfulness itself fosters greater awareness and acceptance of these mental states, providing patients with coping mechanisms to manage stress and improve overall quality of life. This dual focus facilitates a balanced approach to care, addressing the complexity of chronic pain beyond the surface level.

Flexibility in treatment plans, informed by patient feedback, is crucial for improving adherence and outcomes. Pain treatment is rarely linear, and neither should be the strategies employed to manage it. Patients' responses to treatments can vary widely; hence, collecting continuous feedback ensures that interventions remain effective and relevant. Adaptive care models allow for timely modifications based on patient-reported experiences, such as adjusting medication dosages, incorporating new mindfulness techniques, or altering exercise regimens. By aligning treatment adaptations with patient insights, healthcare providers can offer support that resonates well with the current state of the individual's health journey. This adaptability not only prevents stagnation in care but also reinforces trust and cooperation between patients and practitioners.

Education and training play a supportive yet fundamental role in this integrative approach. While the core focus remains on personalized mindfulness integration, ensuring healthcare providers possess adequate knowledge about these techniques is paramount. Training equips them with the skills to guide patients through mindfulness exercises effectively while appreciating the broader implications of mental and emotional well-being in pain management. Providers who are well-versed in mindfulness can tailor interventions more precisely and provide insightful recommendations that empower patients to use mindfulness as a lifelong tool for managing chronic conditions.

Ultimately, combining personalized mindfulness interventions with open communication, holistic assessments, and flexible care plans creates a dynamic framework for chronic pain management. This model respects the individual's lived experience, crafting a healthcare narrative where the person, rather than the pain, takes center stage. It shifts the paradigm from solely treating symptoms to nurturing an inclusive system that recognizes every aspect of health and well-being. As patients engage more deeply with their treatment processes, they not only experience relief from pain but also embark on a journey toward enriched self-awareness and healthier living.

Evaluating Effectiveness of Combined Approaches

Integrating mindfulness with medical treatments is a promising approach for individuals managing chronic pain. To ensure the success of this integration, continuously assessing and refining treatment strategies becomes crucial. Establishing clear assessment metrics not only clarifies goals for patients and providers but also provides a structured foundation for evaluating effectiveness over time. By defining specific, measurable outcomes, healthcare providers can offer more personalized care paths while patients gain a clearer understanding of their progress, fostering a collaborative atmosphere focused on shared goals.

One essential component of this process is gathering patient feedback. Patients' insights are invaluable in highlighting areas that need improvement, as well as understanding how integrated treatments impact resilience. Regularly soliciting feedback through surveys or one-on-one consultations allows healthcare providers to identify trends, customize interventions, and make necessary adjustments. For instance, if patients report increased resilience or decreased reliance on medication after implementing mindfulness practices, it signifies the effectiveness of the integration and encourages further refinement based on real-world results.

Research plays a pivotal role in supporting the validity of integrating mindfulness into traditional medical treatments. Studies have shown that mindfulness can significantly reduce stress and improve overall well-being among patients suffering from chronic conditions (Stange et al., 2014). The evidence-based approach offers credibility and builds confidence among both patients and practitioners. By constantly staying informed about the latest research findings, providers can adapt their strategies to align with proven techniques, ensuring that the benefits of mindfulness are maximized within medical practice.

Continuous evaluation and adjustment of treatment plans are vital for promoting resilience and adaptability. As patients progress, their needs and responses to treatment may change. Ongoing evaluations help detect these changes early, allowing for timely modifications that maintain the relevance and efficacy of the treatment plan. This dynamic approach respects the evolving nature of chronic pain management while empowering patients by involving them in decisions about their care pathways.

An iterative process involving both subjective and objective assessments enhances the efficacy of integrated treatment strategies. Objectively, metrics such as symptom reduction, medication usage, and physical capabilities provide quantifiable data to guide treatment decisions. Subjectively, narratives from patients shed light on personal experiences and challenges, creating a holistic picture that encompasses more than just numbers. Balancing these perspectives ensures that both tangible and intangible elements are considered in strategizing long-term care.

Furthermore, it is crucial to foster environments where open communication and shared learning are encouraged. According to Stange et al. (2014), settings that utilize metrics not punitively but constructively promote innovation and growth. When patients feel safe expressing their experiences and concerns, and when providers listen actively, opportunities for improvement become evident. Collectively, patients and providers can explore which combinations of mindfulness and medical interventions work best, emphasizing long-term effectiveness rather than short-term efficiency.

To support ongoing evaluation effectively, healthcare providers might consider incorporating tools like mindfulness-based exercises specifically designed for monitoring progress. These exercises empower patients to reflect on their mental and physical states regularly, offering insights into how mindfulness affects their condition. Additionally, providers trained in mindfulness techniques can better guide patients, ensuring that adjustments to mindfulness practices are tailored to individual needs while adhering to clinical guidelines (Sheikhrabori et al., 2022).

Insights and Implications

This chapter explored the promising alliance between mindfulness and traditional healthcare, highlighting their combined potential to improve outcomes for individuals managing chronic pain. We delved into how mindfulness practices can enhance physical therapy sessions, offering patients more active roles in their recovery. By listening to patients' unique needs and working alongside them, healthcare providers can cultivate a personalized approach that respects each individual's journey. Facilitating open communication allows both parties to create tailored plans that resonate on personal levels, establishing a partnership founded on understanding and mutual respect.

Additionally, we considered the role of complementary and alternative medicine when integrated with mindfulness, further broadening the spectrum of therapeutic options available.

By fostering this synergy, we touched upon real patient experiences, showing the profound effects of such holistic strategies. The key takeaway is the importance of continuous learning and adjustment, enabling treatments to evolve alongside patients' needs. This dynamic approach not only addresses chronic pain but also cultivates a deeper connection between mind and body, empowering individuals to regain control over their health while nurturing a sense of hope and resilience.

Reference List

CST (she/her), K. E., LCSW, PMH-C. (2023, October 18). *Care Coordination: The Benefits of Collaborative Healthcare*. Wildflower Center for Emotional Health. https://www.wildflowerllc.com/care-coordination-the-benefits-of-collaborative-healthcare/

Chronic Pain and Complementary Health Approaches: Usefulness and Safety. (2023, January). NCCIH; NCCIH. https://www.nccih.nih.gov/health/chronic-pain-and-complementary-health-approaches-usefulness-and-safety

How Home Health Care Professionals Address Chronic Pain. (2025). Regencyhcs.com. https://www.regencyhcs.com/blog/how-home-health-care-professionals-address-chronic-pain?25b4f686_page=5

Hardison, M. E., & Roll, S. C. (2016, April 1). *Mindfulness Interventions in Physical Rehabilitation: A Scoping Review*. American Journal of Occupational Therapy. https://doi.org/10.5014/ajot.2016.018069

Rosen, M. A. (2019). *Teamwork in healthcare: Key discoveries enabling safer, high-quality care.* American Psychologist; NCBI. https://doi.org/10.1037/amp0000298

Stange, K. C., Etz, R. S., Gullett, H., Sweeney, S. A., Miller, W. L., Jaén, C. R., Crabtree, B. F., Nutting, P. A., & Glasgow, R. E. (2014, March 18). *Metrics for Assessing Improvements in Primary Health Care.* Annual Review of Public Health. https://doi.org/10.1146/annurev-publhealth-032013-182438

Sheikhrabori, A., Peyrovi, H., & Khankeh, H. (2022, February 15). *The Main Features of Resilience in Healthcare Providers: A Scoping Review.* Medical Journal of the Islamic Republic of Iran. https://doi.org/10.47176/mjiri.36.3

Themelis, K., & Tang, N. K. Y. (2023, January 1). *The Management of Chronic Pain: Re-Centring Person-Centred Care.* Journal of Clinical Medicine. https://doi.org/10.3390/jcm12226957

Tabish, S. A. (2008). *Complementary and Alternative Healthcare: Is it Evidence-based?* International Journal of Health Sciences. https://pmc.ncbi.nlm.nih.gov/articles/PMC3068720/

Watson, T., Walker, O., Cann, R., & Varghese, A. K. (2022, January 31). *The benefits of mindfulness in mental healthcare professionals.* F1000Research. https://doi.org/10.12688/f1000research.73729.2

CHAPTER 10

Mindfulness and Quality of Life Enhancement

Enhancing one's quality of life through mindfulness is a journey into the present moment, where life's richness is revealed with clarity and appreciation. By aligning our minds and bodies, mindfulness encourages us to engage with life's simple joys and transform mundane experiences into moments of wonder and gratitude. For those living with chronic pain, the practice becomes a gentle invitation to coexist peacefully with discomfort, nurturing a state of being that embraces both mind and body alike. Within this mindful embrace lies the potential for a profound transformation, redefining how individuals perceive their pain and their lives.

This chapter delves into the multifaceted benefits of mindfulness practices as a means to improve overall well-being, particularly for individuals managing chronic pain. Readers will explore how mindfulness can serve as an antidote to the burdens of regret and worry, offering peace in the present, and how gratitude intertwined with mindfulness heightens life satisfaction. The text will also uncover the empowering effects of self-compassion cultivated through mindfulness, relieving self-criticism while fostering emotional resilience. Furthermore, it will highlight the transformative potential of accepting one's present condition, including practical ways to integrate mindfulness seamlessly into daily routines. By highlighting these aspects, the chapter aims to provide readers with the knowledge to harness mindfulness as a pathway to enhance life quality amidst challenges.

Mindfulness and Life Satisfaction

In life, the present moment is like a precious gem often overlooked. Mindfulness, a practice with deep roots, invites us to pause and appreciate these moments as they unfold. It teaches us to see the beauty in everyday experiences, be it the gentle warmth of morning sunlight or the soothing rustle of leaves in the breeze. This connection with the present can lead to a profound sense of fulfillment. When we practice mindfulness, we become more attuned to the small joys that fill our days, and this heightened awareness nurtures feelings of satisfaction and well-being.

Mindfulness also offers an antidote to the burdens of regret and worry. Often, we find ourselves caught in a cycle of dwelling on past mistakes or fretting about future challenges. These thoughts can cloud our minds and dampen our spirits. Through mindfulness, we learn to cultivate acceptance, acknowledging our past without judgment and gently guiding our focus back to the now. This shift in perspective alleviates the weight of regret and diminishes anxiety about what lies ahead. By embracing the present, we can break free from the chains of past grievances and future fears, finding peace in the here and now (Li et al., 2022).

Incorporating gratitude into mindfulness practices further enhances our sense of life satisfaction. Gratitude encourages us to shift our focus from what we lack to the abundance that already exists in our lives. It's about recognizing and appreciating the blessings, big and small, that often go unnoticed. Whether it's a kind word from a friend, the comfort of a warm cup of tea, or the laughter shared with loved ones, gratitude opens our eyes to the richness of our existence. By weaving gratitude into our mindfulness routine, we foster a mindset of appreciation that enriches every aspect of our lives (Crego et al., 2021).

Moreover, mindfulness cultivates self-compassion, a powerful balm for the harsh critic within us all. We often hold ourselves to impossibly high standards, leading to self-criticism and diminished mental health. Mindfulness encourages us to treat ourselves with the same kindness and understanding we would extend to a dear friend. It invites us to embrace our imperfections and recognize that they are part of being human. By nurturing self-compassion, we reduce the sting of self-criticism and create a supportive inner dialogue that promotes emotional resilience and healing.

For individuals grappling with chronic pain, these aspects of mindfulness offer transformative potential. The stress and frustration of living with persistent discomfort can weigh heavily on one's quality of life. Mindfulness provides an alternative approach by encouraging a gentle acceptance of one's current condition. Rather than fighting against the pain, individuals learn to coexist with it, reducing the psychological burden it imposes. This shift in attitude can lead to improved well-being and a more harmonious relationship with their own bodies.

To integrate mindfulness effectively, consider adopting simple yet impactful practices. For instance, guided mindfulness meditations can aid in focusing attention and grounding oneself in the present. A daily gratitude journal can help instill a habit of recognizing the positives in each day. Additionally, regular self-compassion exercises promote a nurturing relationship with oneself. Engaging in these practices regularly can significantly enhance your overall quality of life.

Boosting Energy and Vitality

Mindfulness practices have long been celebrated for their positive impact on enhancing energy levels and overall vitality. By integrating mindfulness into daily life, individuals often find themselves experiencing a remarkable shift in energy and vigor, even amidst the challenges of chronic pain or stress. This transformation stems from several key aspects of mindfulness practices, which promote the balancing of inner resources with external demands.

Firstly, mindful movement, such as yoga or tai chi, demonstrates a powerful synergy between physical activity and mental awareness. These practices encourage participants to engage not just physically but mentally, focusing on each motion and breath. Tai chi, often referred to as "meditation in motion," is particularly effective for this purpose. It harmonizes upper and lower body strength, flexibility, and balance, while simultaneously promoting aerobic conditioning and proprioception — the body's ability to sense its position in space (Harvard Health Publishing, 2022). Regular practice can lead to enhanced vitality, as it fosters a profound connection between mind and body, ultimately invigorating one's entire being.

Similarly, yoga combines physical postures, breathing exercises, and meditation to amplify energy levels. The slow, deliberate movements coupled with focused breathing help increase blood flow and oxygen supply throughout the body, rejuvenating both muscles and mind. Such practices enable practitioners to cultivate an internal reservoir of energy that can be drawn upon during times of need, thereby fostering resilience and sustained vitality.

In addition to physical movement, taking structured mindfulness breaks serves a crucial role in replenishing energy reserves. Amidst busy days dominated by high-pressure tasks, short intermissions dedicated to mindfulness can prevent burnout. These breaks involve stepping away from pressing tasks, closing one's eyes, and focusing on deep breaths or a brief body scan. Such mindful pauses allow the mind to reset, refocus, and recharge, subsequently boosting productivity and mental clarity. This simple yet effective strategy ensures that energy levels remain consistent, and cognitive functions are maintained at their peak.

Moreover, mindfulness nurtures conscious lifestyle choices that significantly impact energy levels. When individuals become more attuned to their bodies and minds through mindfulness, they are naturally inclined towards healthier habits. For example, mindfulness encourages better eating patterns by fostering awareness of hunger cues and satiety, deterring emotional eating, and promoting nutrition-conscious decisions. Similarly, improved sleep hygiene becomes attainable as mindfulness teaches relaxation techniques, helping the body prepare for rest and improving overall sleep quality. By embracing these habits, individuals create a foundation for sustained energy and vitality.

Furthermore, enhanced focus achieved through mindfulness leads to sharper mental clarity and more efficient task completion. Mindfulness cultivates an ability to concentrate on the present moment without distraction, filtering out unnecessary stimuli that drain mental resources. This heightened concentration enables individuals to manage their workloads more effectively, completing tasks with greater precision and less fatigue. By reducing mental clutter, mindfulness opens up pathways to innovative thinking, problem-solving, and creative exploration, all of which contribute to an individual's overall sense of vitality.

Guidelines for incorporating mindfulness into daily routines vary depending on individual preferences and needs, yet the core principle remains consistent: intentionality. To begin, engaging in regular sessions of mindful movement like yoga or tai chi is advisable. Allocating specific times of day for these activities ensures consistency and maximizes benefits. Similarly, scheduling mindfulness breaks strategically throughout the day can keep energy levels stable. It might involve setting reminders to take five-minute breathing exercises during work or incorporating a short meditative walk after lunch.

Conscious lifestyle changes, guided by mindfulness, are another area where guidelines prove beneficial. Individuals can start by keeping a food journal to associate feelings of energy or exhaustion with dietary choices. Similarly, exploring mindfulness-based approaches to enhance sleep, like maintaining a consistent bedtime routine, can offer substantial improvements. Consulting with a healthcare professional or mindfulness coach may provide additional structure and personalized guidance.

Improving Sleep Quality

The impact of mindfulness on enhancing sleep quality and restfulness is profound, offering a natural alternative to pharmaceutical solutions. Mindfulness relaxation techniques, particularly deep breathing and body scans, are powerful tools for signaling the body to wind down before sleep. These practices help individuals focus on their breath or the physical sensations in their body, allowing them to relax and disengage from the day's stresses. The process of slowing down the breath can trigger the parasympathetic nervous system, which reduces stress hormones and prepares the body for a restful night. In essence, these techniques serve as a gentle cue for both mind and body to transition into a state of restfulness.

Increasing awareness of thoughts through mindfulness also plays a critical role in managing nighttime anxiety and mental chatter. Mindfulness teaches individuals to observe their thoughts without judgment, thereby reducing the intensity of worry that often amplifies during quiet nighttime hours. By acknowledging thoughts as they arise and gently redirecting focus back to the present moment—for instance, by concentrating on the rhythm of the breath—a person can prevent spirals of anxiety that disrupt the onset of sleep. This practice allows the mind to settle, creating a mental environment conducive to falling asleep more easily.

Mindfulness significantly promotes better sleep hygiene by encouraging healthier pre-sleep activities and routines. Sleep hygiene refers to habits and practices that are beneficial for sleeping well on a regular basis. Mindful individuals become more attuned to the impact of activities such as screen time and late-night snacking on their sleep patterns. Consequently, they are more likely to adopt beneficial pre-sleep practices like dimming lights, reading, or engaging in calming activities that support the body's natural preparation for sleep. This heightened awareness helps cultivate an evening routine that enhances the likelihood of achieving quality rest.

Furthermore, engaging in mindfulness meditation directly improves sleep quality and helps reduce symptoms of insomnia. Research has indicated that mindfulness interventions can lead to significant improvements in sleep quality compared to nonspecific active controls (Rusch et al., 2018). Participants who practice mindfulness meditation experience decreased arousal levels, as meditation reduces psychological and physiological distress that otherwise fuels insomnia. As a result, those struggling with sleep disturbances, including those with chronic pain conditions seeking alternative methods for pain management, can find relief through consistent mindfulness practice.

Guidelines for incorporating mindfulness into daily routines can be helpful. For relaxation techniques, consider setting aside a dedicated time each evening for deep breathing exercises or a body scan. This practice can be brief—perhaps just five to ten minutes—but it's important to create a calm environment free of distractions to maximize its effectiveness. For managing sleep disruptors, practice observing your thoughts throughout the day as a way to build awareness. When anxious thoughts emerge at night, use this skill to guide your attention back to the present moment, perhaps by focusing on the gentleness of your breath.

To improve sleep hygiene, practice mindful technology use. Set limits on screen time before bed, and consider implementing a digital detox in the hour leading up to sleep. Instead, engage in mindful reading or listen to calming music. Establishing a consistent sleep schedule is another effective strategy; try going to bed and waking at the same times each day to regulate your body's internal clock. Lastly, for mindfulness meditation, beginners might start with guided meditations available through various apps or online resources. Choose a comfortable position and dedicate a few moments to focus on your breath, gradually increasing the duration as you become more comfortable with the practice.

Social Connectedness

In today's fast-paced world, where connections can feel fleeting and loneliness often looms, mindfulness emerges as a beacon for enhancing social bonds. By fostering empathy, improving communication skills, combating isolation, and building communities, mindfulness offers valuable tools for enriching our interactions with others.

Empathy development stands at the forefront of mindfulness benefits. When we practice being present and attentive to our own experiences, we become more attuned to the nuances of others' emotions and perspectives. This heightened empathy allows us to connect on a deeper level, understanding not just the words spoken but the emotions behind them. Through mindfulness, we cultivate compassion and a genuine desire to understand the experiences of those around us. This understanding fosters stronger social connections and diminishes feelings of isolation.

Communication is a cornerstone of relationships, and mindfulness plays a crucial role in enhancing active listening skills. By centering ourselves and focusing wholly on the present moment, we learn to listen without interrupting or mentally preparing our responses. This shift in approach leads to more meaningful conversations, where both parties feel heard and valued. Mindful listening encourages us to fully engage with the speaker, establishing trust and improving relationship dynamics.

It transforms ordinary exchanges into opportunities for deeper connection and understanding.

Combatting loneliness is another significant area where mindfulness proves beneficial. Loneliness often stems from a sense of disconnection from oneself and others. Mindfulness helps individuals recognize their internal states, allowing them to acknowledge feelings of loneliness without judgment. This self-awareness opens the door to understanding that these feelings are part of the human experience, shared by many. By embracing our own vulnerability, we become more open to connecting with others, reducing the emotional distance that loneliness creates.

Furthermore, participating in group mindfulness activities provides opportunities for social interaction and shared experiences. Group sessions offer a sense of belonging, where individuals can connect with others who share similar interests and challenges. These gatherings create a supportive environment where participants can explore mindfulness together, reinforcing communal ties. The collective energy and motivation derived from practicing mindfulness in a group setting can enhance individual commitment and persistence in mindful practices (Sutton, 2020).

Effective guidelines for improving active listening through mindfulness include focusing entirely on the speaker, maintaining eye contact, and acknowledging what is said with nods or brief verbal affirmations. Reflective listening, where you paraphrase the speaker's points to confirm understanding, also deepens engagement. Practicing these techniques regularly can transform everyday interactions into more rewarding experiences.

Mindfulness reduces loneliness by encouraging recognition of our shared humanity. By accepting our feelings and the impermanent nature of emotions, we can dismantle the barriers loneliness erects. Mindfulness teaches us to be gentle with ourselves, and this acceptance allows us to reach out to others, creating bonds that alleviate isolation. Participation in group mindfulness activities further strengthens these connections. Engaging in such activities not only provides a shared mindfulness journey but also nurtures a network of support and understanding among peers.

Building community through mindfulness emphasizes the importance of inclusivity and shared purpose. Whether it's a meditation group meeting regularly or a mindfulness-based workshop, these community-centric initiatives offer a platform for individuals to come together, learn from one another, and grow collectively. They foster an environment where participants are encouraged to share their experiences and insights, enhancing communal ties and creating a supportive network that extends beyond the activity itself.

The impact of these mindfulness practices extends beyond individual benefits, influencing broader social outcomes. Research supports the idea that mindfulness interventions can mitigate feelings of loneliness and isolation by promoting acceptance and equanimity towards social interactions (Lindsay et al., 2019). This acceptance leads to more frequent and diverse social contacts, ultimately strengthening social networks and enhancing community well-being.

Mindfulness and Personal Growth

Mindfulness is a practice that extends beyond mere relaxation; it serves as a catalyst for personal growth and development. By fostering self-awareness, mindfulness empowers individuals to delve deep into their inner landscapes, unlocking insights into their values, aspirations, and goals. This journey of self-discovery allows people to cultivate a more authentic connection with themselves, enabling them to identify what truly matters in life.

The self-awareness journey facilitated by mindfulness involves observing one's thoughts and emotions without judgment. Through practices like meditation and reflection, individuals learn to tune into their internal dialogue, discerning patterns that may have previously gone unnoticed. For instance, during mindful breathing exercises, one might become aware of recurring thoughts about a particular career path or relationship, prompting them to explore these areas further. By paying attention to the present moment, mindfulness aids individuals in unveiling hidden desires and ambitions, thereby promoting personal growth aligned with genuine values and long-term objectives.

Resilience is another significant benefit of mindfulness, crucial for navigating the complexities of life. Mindfulness encourages a flexible mindset, a vital component for overcoming challenges. When faced with obstacles, a mindful approach promotes creative problem-solving and adaptability, allowing individuals to view setbacks as opportunities for growth rather than insurmountable barriers. The practice of mindfulness fosters resilience by helping people detach from immediate emotional reactions and approach problems with a calm and composed demeanor (Marano, 2023).

For example, consider someone dealing with chronic pain. Through mindfulness, they may learn to observe their pain without letting it define their day-to-day existence. Instead of succumbing to frustration or despair, mindfulness encourages exploring alternative coping strategies, such as visualization techniques or mindful movement. By reframing their experience, they build resilience, enhance their quality of life, and learn to thrive despite ongoing challenges.

Mindfulness also cultivates a mindset of curiosity and continuous learning. By encouraging individuals to remain open and receptive to new experiences, mindfulness enriches personal development journeys. Embracing a curious mindset often leads to discovering unexplored interests, facilitating adaptability in an ever-changing world. This openness encourages lifelong learning, as the quest for knowledge becomes an intrinsic motivator for growth.

Consider how mindfulness can transform mundane daily experiences into opportunities for discovery. While walking in nature, for example, a person practicing mindful awareness may notice details they previously overlooked—the interplay of light and shadow, subtle fragrances, or the chorus of birds. These observations foster curiosity about the natural world and instill a desire for further exploration. Mindfulness nudges individuals toward embracing novelty, leading to new hobbies, skills, or even career paths that align with evolving interests (What Is the Best Form of Personal Development, 2024).

Furthermore, mindfulness invites intentional goal setting and reflection, essential components of meaningful personal development. When individuals engage in mindfulness practices, they create space for thoughtful consideration of their life's direction. This intentionality paves the way for mindful decision-making, rooted in personal values and priorities.

Setting mindful goals involves tuning into both short-term desires and long-term aspirations. For example, someone passionate about environmental sustainability may set small, actionable goals to reduce waste, while also nurturing larger visions of influencing policy change. Regular reflection sessions can serve as checkpoints, enabling individuals to assess progress and make necessary adjustments. This cycle of goal setting, action, and reflection ensures alignment with evolving values and fosters a sense of fulfillment in personal pursuits.

Guiding this process are simple yet powerful questions: What truly matters to me? How can I honor my values through my everyday actions? Engaging with these inquiries fosters a deeper understanding of oneself and one's path, empowering individuals to navigate life's complexities with clarity and purpose.

As individuals embark on their mindfulness journey, it's essential to incorporate goal check-ins into their routines. Regularly reviewing personal development goals helps maintain focus and motivation, ensuring that efforts align with overarching objectives. Celebrating milestones along the way reinforces positive behavior and propels further growth. When progress feels challenging, it's helpful to remember that each small step contributes to a broader tapestry of personal growth.

Mindfulness, with its emphasis on remaining present, serves as a gentle reminder that personal development is a continuous, lifelong journey. It encourages individuals to embrace imperfection and view setbacks as valuable teachers rather than failures. By incorporating mindfulness into daily life, individuals can cultivate resilience, curiosity, and intentionality, creating a fertile ground for ongoing transformation.

Insights and Implications

Mindfulness practices, embraced with empathy and creativity, empower individuals to improve their overall well-being, especially those navigating chronic pain. By focusing on the present moment, mindfulness encourages a deeper appreciation for life's small joys and nurtures gratitude. This shift in perspective helps lift the burdens of past regrets and future anxieties, fostering a profound sense of satisfaction. Engaging regularly in mindfulness exercises like guided meditations or keeping a gratitude journal can unveil new layers of self-awareness. These simple yet impactful routines enable people to see beauty in daily life, enriching their journey towards better mental health.

Furthermore, mindfulness integrates seamlessly with other aspects of self-care, creating a harmonious lifestyle supporting energy, vitality, and restful sleep. Mindful movement practices, such as yoga or tai chi, offer a dynamic blend of physical engagement and mental focus that invigorates both body and soul. Meanwhile, structured mindfulness breaks and mindful bedtime routines help replenish energy reserves and ease the mind into restful slumber. By weaving these habits into daily life, individuals can cultivate a balanced rhythm that nurtures resilience and supports their pursuit of personal growth and healing. Embracing mindfulness opens new pathways to thrive in spite of challenges, allowing anyone to live fully and meaningfully.

Reference List

Crego, A., Yela, J. R., Gómez-Martínez, M. Á., Riesco-Matías, P., & Petisco-Rodríguez, C. (2021, January 21). *Relationships between Mindfulness, Purpose in Life, Happiness, Anxiety, and Depression: Testing a Mediation Model in a Sample of Women*. International Journal of Environmental Research and Public Health. https://doi.org/10.3390/ijerph18030925

Harvard Health Publishing. (2022, May 24). *The health benefits of tai chi*. Harvard Health; Harvard Health. https://www.health.harvard.edu/staying-healthy/the-health-benefits-of-tai-chi

Li, X., Ma, L., & Li, Q. (2022, June 30). *How Mindfulness Affects Life Satisfaction: Based on the Mindfulness-to-Meaning Theory*. Frontiers in Psychology. https://doi.org/10.3389/fpsyg.2022.887940

Lindsay, E. K., Young, S., Brown, K. W., Smyth, J. M., & Creswell, J. D. (2019, February 11). *Mindfulness training reduces loneliness and increases social contact in a randomized controlled trial*. Proceedings of the National Academy of Sciences. https://doi.org/10.1073/pnas.1813588116

Marano, S. (2023, July 10). *Pathway to Growth - How Personal Growth Will Change Your Life*. LSC. https://www.lavenderskycounselling.com/post/personal-growth-how-personal-growth-will-change-your-life

Rusch, H. L., Rosario, M., Levison, L. M., Olivera, A., Livingston, W. S., Wu, T., & Gill, J. M. (2018, December 21). *The effect of mindfulness meditation on sleep quality: a systematic review and meta-analysis of randomized controlled trials*. Annals of the New York Academy of Sciences. https://doi.org/10.1111/nyas.13996

Sutton, J. (2020, July 24). *Practicing Mindfulness in Groups: 9 Activities and Exercises*. PositivePsychology.com. https://positivepsychology.com/group-mindfulness-activities/

Team, B. E. (2024, March 4). *Boost Energy Levels With The Mind-Body Connection | BetterHelp*. Betterhelp.com; BetterHelp. https://www.betterhelp.com/advice/how-to/how-to-boost-energy-levels-through-the-mind-body-connection/

What is the Best Form of Personal Development. (2024). Morningcoach.com. https://www.morningcoach.com/blog/whatisthebestforofpersonaldevelopment

CHAPTER 11

Role of Caregivers in Mindfulness Practices

Caregivers play a vital role in introducing mindfulness practices to those experiencing chronic pain. Mindfulness, characterized by being present and non-judgmental, offers caregivers an empowering tool to enhance both their well-being and that of the individuals they support. This chapter delves into the intricate world where mindfulness practices are not just self-care techniques but bridges connecting caregivers with those they care for. In exploring the transformative impact of mindfulness on caregiving, we gain insight into how these simple practices can cultivate an environment of calmness and understanding.

In this chapter, caregivers will embark on a journey of discovering various strategies to incorporate mindfulness seamlessly into their routines. Readers will explore how community resources and online support groups provide a network of encouragement and shared experiences. Through professional counseling and peer mentorship, caregivers find avenues to contextualize and navigate their emotional landscapes. The discussion also covers practical mindfulness techniques tailored to fit individual pain conditions, allowing for personalized care. Furthermore, it touches upon the importance of balancing caregiver duties with mindfulness practices, emphasizing the need for strategic time management and setting boundaries, thereby creating a sustainable caregiving model. By aligning intentions and fostering feedback mechanisms within caregiver-patient relationships, the chapter illustrates how mindfulness not only assists in managing stress but also strengthens empathetic connections. Thus, this exploration opens doors for caregivers seeking to deepen their understanding and enrich their interactions—ultimately benefiting both themselves and those entrusted to their care.

Caregiver Support Systems

In the demanding world of caregiving, a robust support system is fundamental for caregivers navigating their mindfulness journey. By fostering connections and gaining insights, these systems can significantly enhance caregivers' well-being and the quality of care they provide.

Community resources act as an essential pillar in cultivating such support systems. Local community centers, libraries, or wellness programs often host sessions that bring caregivers together, creating a sense of belonging and camaraderie. These resources help alleviate the feeling of isolation that many caregivers experience. As one caregiver noted, joining a local group helped them forge lifelong friendships, emphasizing that shared experiences cultivate deeper relationships (C, mentor). Participating in community events not only offers companionship but introduces caregivers to new mindfulness techniques. Learning alongside peers provides diverse perspectives and helps tailor practices to specific needs (D, PS).

Moreover, online support groups have emerged as invaluable platforms for caregivers. The digital realm offers flexibility, allowing caregivers to connect with others regardless of geographic constraints. This virtual environment serves as a stage for sharing experiences and advice, often under the guidance of experts who specialize in mindfulness practices. Participants gain access to valuable knowledge and encouragement, critical components in effectively managing stress and maintaining emotional resilience. One source highlighted, "People realize there is somewhere you're not the outcast... It's okay to talk about anything" (B, PL), emphasizing the inclusive nature of online communities. Caregivers benefit from broadening their understanding while feeling supported in a non-judgmental space.

Professional counseling also plays a crucial role in supporting caregivers by normalizing their emotional experiences. Engaging with counselors helps caregivers contextualize their emotions, increasing self-awareness, and promoting emotional health. This process not only validates their feelings but empowers them to better handle the emotional toll of caregiving. Counseling sessions offer a safe environment where caregivers can candidly discuss challenges without fear of judgment, leading to improved mental health outcomes (Joo et al., 2022). Ultimately, this heightened awareness fosters more empathetic interactions with those in pain.

Peer mentoring introduces another layer of support, particularly beneficial for novice caregivers. Experienced caregivers impart practical advice born from firsthand experiences, providing mentees with insights into effective mindfulness strategies. Such mentorship arrangements encourage a two-way exchange of knowledge, invigorating both parties with fresh perspectives on mindfulness practices. One source shared how role modeling offers inspiration, noting, "You see someone who's just like you... achieve" (B, PL). This illustrates the motivational impact of peer support, highlighting its ability to foster resilience and innovation among caregivers.

While exploring these support systems, it's vital to remember that each caregiver's journey is unique. Guidelines for building strong community resources suggest organizing regular meetings at varied times, ensuring accessibility and accommodating different schedules. Encouraging open communication within these groups enhances trust and facilitates collaboration among members. Furthermore, investing time in understanding online networks allows caregivers to identify suitable groups that align with their mindfulness goals. Engagement in professional counseling should focus on consistency, enabling caregivers to establish rapport with their therapists over time.

Teaching Mindfulness Techniques

In the journey of caregiving, mindfulness emerges as a profound ally for both caregivers and those they support. By introducing basic mindfulness exercises that are simple yet impactful, caregivers can create an environment where they and their patients feel more at ease. Mindfulness is not about emptying the mind but focusing on the present moment without judgment. Techniques such as deep breathing, mindful listening, or grounding exercises foster an atmosphere of calm and connection. Caregivers can encourage both themselves and their patients to engage in short, guided sessions where each person focuses on their breath, noting the air flowing in and out, allowing the body to relax (Mayo Clinic Staff, 2022).

Customizing mindfulness techniques to align with individual pain conditions further strengthens the caregiver-patient relationship. Acknowledging that each person's experience of pain is unique invites a level of empathy that enhances connection. For instance, a patient dealing with chronic back pain might find a seated meditation more comfortable than lying flat for a body scan exercise. As activities are tailored to meet specific needs, patients often feel heard and validated, which can lead to greater emotional comfort and engagement in their care.

Caregiver burnout is a significant risk when managing the constant demands of looking after others. Mindfulness provides essential tools for stress relief, reducing feelings of overwhelm and fostering resilience. Stress-relief techniques like progressive muscle relaxation or visualization enable caregivers to unwind, offering moments of tranquility in their busy day. By incorporating mindfulness into daily routines, caregivers not only rejuvenate themselves but also improve the quality of care they provide. The act of mindfulness itself becomes a refuge, a few minutes of peace amid the chaos of caregiving (American Cancer Society, 2020).

Engagement strategies are crucial for motivating participation from those under a caregiver's care, thereby fostering a sense of agency and autonomy. Taking time to explain the benefits of mindfulness to patients, perhaps through sharing simple success stories or demonstrating exercises together, encourages active involvement. For example, inviting a patient to participate in a mindful walk around the garden, where they note what they see, hear, and smell, can transform the exercise into a shared exploration. As caregivers and patients engage in these practices together, it strengthens trust and cooperation, making the therapeutic process more collaborative and less hierarchical.

The integration of mindfulness exercises into caregiving routines doesn't require substantial changes or additional time commitments. Simple activities, such as pausing for a moment before starting a task or practicing gratitude during daily routines, can be seamlessly woven into the day. This approach ensures that mindfulness remains accessible and manageable, preventing it from becoming another duty that overwhelms already stretched caregivers.

Furthermore, by cultivating a mindful presence, caregivers model behaviors that patients can mirror, creating a ripple effect of calmness and attentiveness. Patients observe and learn how these small shifts towards mindfulness can have a big impact on their own lives, empowering them with tools to better manage their experiences of pain and discomfort.

Ultimately, the inclusion of mindfulness techniques empowers caregivers by providing a sustainable way to navigate the complexities of their role. These practices offer more than just temporary relief; they open a pathway to deeper understanding and acceptance of the present moment. In this way, caregivers are better equipped to respond with compassion and patience, qualities that enrich their interactions with those in their care.

Emotional Resilience for Caregivers

In the challenging landscape of caregiving, especially for those dealing with chronic pain, building emotional resilience is not just beneficial—it's essential. As caregivers navigate their roles, they face unique stressors that can take a toll on their emotional well-being. This section delves into strategies that empower caregivers to cultivate emotional resilience, thereby improving their ability to support others effectively.

Self-compassion is a cornerstone in mitigating stress and boosting caregiving efficiency. It involves treating oneself with the same kindness and understanding as one would offer a friend. Dr. Kristin Neff's work highlights self-compassion practices as powerful tools for reducing burnout and enhancing caregiver performance (Neff, 2024). Embracing these practices can make a remarkable difference; they help caregivers acknowledge their struggles without judgment, fostering an environment where they can recharge emotionally and approach their duties with renewed vigor.

Tailoring stress management techniques is another critical component. Stress management isn't one-size-fits-all, so caregivers benefit from customizing methods to suit their individual needs and circumstances. Whether through meditation, exercise, or creative outlets like journaling, personalized approaches provide targeted relief. By identifying what truly alleviates stress, caregivers can bolster their emotional resilience amidst demanding situations (Self-Care Begins with Self-Compassion, 2025). A mindful pause can be a simple yet effective technique—taking moments throughout the day to breathe deeply and center oneself can reduce tension and improve focus.

Routine mindful reflection serves as a guiding light, helping caregivers better understand their emotions and navigate their experiences. Engaging in practices such as noting meditation, which develops awareness of thoughts and emotions, empowers caregivers to observe their feelings without becoming overwhelmed (Neff, 2024). This practice allows them to process emotions constructively, setting the stage for thoughtful decision-making and future actions. Consistently reflecting on daily experiences results in increased emotional clarity, enabling caregivers to identify patterns and adapt their strategies accordingly.

Establishing boundaries is vital for protecting emotional energy and ensuring sustainable caregiving. Caregivers often feel compelled to give endlessly, but without boundaries, they risk emotional exhaustion and burnout. Boundaries create a necessary buffer zone, allowing caregivers to maintain their own well-being while fulfilling their responsibilities. Setting limits on time and tasks ensures that caregivers do not overextend themselves, preserving their capacity to care effectively over the long term (Self-Care Begins with Self-Compassion, 2025). By communicating their needs clearly and asserting their limits compassionately, caregivers foster healthier relationships both personally and professionally.

To further support these strategies, mindfulness basics offer additional tools to reinforce emotional resilience. Mindfulness encourages present-moment awareness and acceptance, providing caregivers with skills to manage stress before it becomes overwhelming. Practices like affectionate breathing or a compassionate body scan gently redirect attention and cultivate a sense of peace, even in challenging times (Neff, 2024). Integrating mindfulness into daily routines can transform caregiving from a source of stress into an opportunity for personal growth.

Adapting techniques for individual circumstances emphasizes the importance of flexibility in caregiving strategies. Each caregiving situation is unique, requiring caregivers to adjust their approaches to meet specific needs. For instance, if one method of stress relief proves ineffective, being open to trying new ones is crucial. This adaptability enhances emotional resilience by encouraging caregivers to remain responsive rather than rigid, allowing for continuous improvement in their caregiving roles (Self-Care Begins with Self-Compassion, 2025).

Incorporating these strategies into a caregiver's routine doesn't happen overnight. It's a gradual process that requires patience and persistence. However, by consciously prioritizing emotional resilience through self-compassion, tailored stress management, mindful reflection, and boundary-setting, caregivers can nurture their own well-being while providing exceptional support to those they care for. They become not only providers of care but also models of resilience and strength, demonstrating that nurturing oneself is as crucial as nurturing others.

Creating a Mindfulness Partnership

Establishing a collaborative mindfulness relationship between caregivers and patients can profoundly impact their journey together, fostering both engagement and emotional connection. As caregivers begin to weave mindfulness practices into the care process, joint mindfulness sessions emerge as a cornerstone for promoting mutual engagement and trust. These sessions create an environment where both parties actively participate in meditative exercises, strengthening their bond through shared experiences. By engaging together, caregivers and patients build trust, as each session becomes a safe space for communication and understanding. Trust, once established, serves as a foundation for open dialogue and deeper connections, enabling more personalized and effective care.

Setting shared intentions plays a crucial role in aligning expectations between caregivers and patients. When both parties voice their intentions, they develop a unified vision of what mindfulness practice means within their relationship. This alignment reduces anxiety, as individuals feel assured that their goals and aspirations are understood and respected. A sense of teamwork flourishes, creating a cooperative dynamic that enhances the caregiving experience. Patients, who often face anxiety from uncertainty and change, find solace in knowing that their caregivers are aligned with their needs and interests. For caregivers, this alignment provides reassurance that they are effectively supporting their patients' well-being, leading to more meaningful interactions.

To ensure that mindfulness sessions are beneficial, feedback mechanisms should be integrated into the process. Incorporating structured feedback encourages transparency, allowing caregivers to adjust mindfulness techniques based on individual patient responses. Regular feedback fosters adaptability, ensuring that the practices remain relevant and effective. Caregivers can introduce simple methods for exchanging thoughts and observations, such as regularly asking patients how they felt after a session or if they have any suggestions for future activities. This ongoing dialogue not only refines the practices but also empowers patients by giving them a voice in their care, enhancing their engagement and commitment to the process.

Another vital aspect of a collaborative mindfulness relationship is celebrating progress. Recognizing and acknowledging milestones, no matter how small, strengthens bonds and fuels continuous practice. Celebrations can be as simple as expressing appreciation, sharing joyful moments, or reflecting on positive changes noticed over time. These moments of acknowledgment reinforce the feeling of accomplishment, encouraging both caregivers and patients to remain committed to their mindfulness journey. For patients, especially those battling chronic pain or cognitive challenges, these celebrations boost morale, offering tangible evidence of progress and hope. Caregivers benefit too, as recognizing progress reminds them of their impactful role, providing motivation and satisfaction in their caregiving duties.

Implementing guidelines for engagement strategies can facilitate the initial stages of a mindfulness relationship. Simple actions, like creating a comfortable setting and establishing routine schedules for practice, can significantly enhance engagement levels. Over time, integrating self-compassion into mindfulness sessions allows caregivers and patients to approach challenges with kindness and patience. Encouraging self-compassion can mitigate feelings of frustration and helplessness, replacing them with understanding and patience. Caregivers can lead by example, demonstrating self-compassion through their interactions, which in turn encourages patients to adopt similar attitudes towards themselves.

Stress management is another domain where mindfulness shines, providing tools to handle the emotional strain associated with caregiving and chronic illness. Techniques such as deep breathing or guided meditation can alleviate stress, benefiting both parties. Regular practice of these techniques can lower cortisol levels, reducing the physical manifestations of stress and contributing to better health outcomes for both caregivers and patients. Implementing stress management techniques promotes emotional balance, essential for maintaining a nurturing caregiving environment.

Mindful reflection serves as a valuable tool for facilitating personal growth and insight within the caregiver-patient dynamic. Setting aside time for reflection after sessions encourages both parties to consider the emotional and cognitive impacts of the practices. Caregivers might reflect on their approach and effectiveness, while patients can contemplate shifts in their mood or mindset. Establishing dedicated reflection periods fosters an atmosphere of continuous learning and improvement, empowering both parties to refine their mindfulness practices further.

Balancing Caregiver Responsibilities

Balancing caregiving duties with personal mindfulness practices requires thoughtful strategies, particularly in managing time efficiently. For caregivers, time management is crucial but often challenging due to unpredictable schedules and numerous responsibilities. To prioritize mindfulness within such a busy agenda, it's beneficial to set aside specific times for mindfulness activities and stick to this schedule as consistently as possible. Utilizing tools like planners or mobile apps can assist in visualizing these slots, ensuring they remain fixed despite the day-to-day chaos. Even small pockets of time, like a few minutes before bedtime or early morning, can offer valuable moments for reflection and stress relief.

In addition to individual time-management efforts, delegating responsibilities is another key strategy that significantly alleviates stress. Many caregivers feel compelled to handle every aspect of care, but reaching out for help creates opportunities for shared effort and collaboration. This can involve enlisting family members or friends for support with specific tasks or tapping into community resources available for caregivers. By spreading the responsibilities, caregivers create space not only for their personal well-being but also foster a more cooperative and cohesive care environment. This delegation allows them to focus on quality interactions and care rather than being overwhelmed by endless lists of tasks.

Incorporating mindfulness into daily routines turns mundane chores into opportunities for self-care. Mindfulness doesn't require special settings or lengthy periods; instead, it can be seamlessly integrated into everyday activities. Simple acts, like focusing on the process of washing dishes or the sensations felt during a walk, transform regular tasks into mindful practices. This approach encourages caregivers to remain present and engaged, enhancing both mental clarity and emotional resilience. Routine activities become less of a chore and more of an opportunity to connect with the present, providing much-needed breaks from the whirlwind of caregiving demands.

Regular self-check-ins are vital for maintaining awareness of one's own well-being. They act as pauses throughout the day for caregivers to evaluate their mental and physical state, offering insights into any necessary adjustments needed to maintain balance. This practice prevents burnout by fostering an ongoing conversation with oneself about needs and limitations. Checking in can be as simple as taking a few deep breaths and asking how one feels or identifying areas of tension or stress. This consistent self-awareness promotes proactive steps toward self-care, whether by adjusting workloads or dedicating additional time to relaxation.

Implementing these strategies demands setting boundaries that protect personal time without compromising caregiving duties. Clearly defined limits on what tasks are manageable ensure that caregivers do not become overextended. By saying no to overwhelming obligations when necessary, caregivers safeguard their health and efficiency. Setting boundaries may initially seem challenging, but it cultivates a sustainable routine where both caregivers' and patients' needs are equally respected and met. These checks can also guide decision-making processes regarding commitments, ensuring energy is allocated appropriately between caregiving and self-care.

For balance to be effectively achieved, engaging in joint mindfulness sessions with those cared for can also be valuable. When caregivers and patients practice mindfulness together, it strengthens their bond and enhances mutual understanding. These shared moments provide a peaceful context for collaboration, reducing anxiety and fostering teamwork, which can enrich the caregiving relationship through empathy and shared goals.

Moreover, setting shared intentions at the start of these joint sessions can align expectations between caregivers and their loved ones. Such alignment reduces misunderstandings and instills a sense of unity in pursuit of shared wellness goals. Feedback mechanisms further ensure that these practices remain adaptable and effective, allowing caregivers to respond to the evolving needs of both themselves and those they care for. Embracing openness to feedback helps refine mindfulness techniques, tailoring them to maximize benefits and engagement.

Final Thoughts

In this chapter, we've explored the vital role mindfulness plays in caregiving, particularly for those experiencing chronic pain. We've examined how caregivers can utilize various support systems like community groups, online platforms, and professional counseling to enhance their mindfulness journey. These resources help caregivers feel less isolated and more empowered as they navigate the complexities of caring for others. By incorporating mindfulness techniques into everyday routines, caregivers can find moments of peace, build emotional resilience, and maintain balance in their demanding roles. This structured approach not only alleviates stress but also deepens the caregiver-patient connection, creating a supportive environment for healing.

Caregivers who practice mindfulness aren't just helping themselves; they are creating an uplifting experience for their patients as well. Joint participation in mindfulness exercises promotes trust and understanding, making the therapeutic process collaborative and enriching. As each caregiver finds unique ways to manage stress, set boundaries, and engage with their patients, they pave the way for meaningful and compassionate interactions. Through consistent application of these practices, caregivers become resilient allies in the journey toward managing chronic pain, illustrating that small mindful changes can lead to significant improvements in the quality of care and life for everyone involved.

Reference List

(2022). Sambaathome.com. https://www.sambaathome.com/blog/supporting-family-caregivers?ca2cba62_page=11

American Cancer Society. (2020, December 2). *Practice Mindfulness and Relaxation*. Www.cancer.org. https://www.cancer.org/cancer/survivorship/coping/practice-mindfulness-and-relaxation.html

Balancing Caregiving Responsibilities with Self-Care: Tips for a Healthier, Happier You. (2025, January 13). BeatCancer. https://beatcancer.eu/resources/psychosocial-care/article/balancing-caregiving-responsibilities-with-self-care/

Innis, A. D., Tolea, M. I., & Galvin, J. E. (2021, January 1). *The Effect of Baseline Patient and Caregiver Mindfulness on Dementia Outcomes.* Journal of Alzheimer's Disease. https://doi.org/10.3233/JAD-201292

Joo, J. H., Bone, L., Forte, J., Kirley, E., Lynch, T., & Aboumatar, H. (2022). *The benefits and challenges of established peer support programmes for patients, informal caregivers, and healthcare providers.* Family Practice. https://doi.org/10.1093/fampra/cmac004

Mayo Clinic Staff. (2022, October 11). *Mindfulness exercises.* Mayo Clinic. https://www.mayoclinic.org/healthy-lifestyle/consumer-health/in-depth/mindfulness-exercises/art-20046356

Neff, K. (2024). *Self-compassion practices.* Self-Compassion. https://self-compassion.org/self-compassion-practices/

Senior Lifestyle. (2025, February 11). *Mindfulness for Caregivers: Cultivating Presence and Resilience in Daily Life.* Senior Lifestyle. https://www.seniorlifestyle.com/resources/blog/mindfulness-for-caregivers-cultivating-presence-and-resilience-in-daily-life/

Self-Care Begins with Self-Compassion. (2025). Caregiving.com. https://www.caregiving.com/content/self-compassion-for-caregivers

\r\n   \n   *The Benefits Of Mindfulness Practices For Dementia Patients\n   \r\n.* (2022). Assuredassistedliving.com. https://www.assuredassistedliving.com/the-benefits-of-mindfulness-practices-for-dementia-patients

CHAPTER 12

Community and Support Networks

Building supportive networks for mindfulness practice can be a lifeline for individuals dealing with chronic pain. Engaging in mindfulness within a community setting fosters an environment rich in empathy and shared understanding, where individuals find encouragement to persevere in their practice. As people come together with mutual goals, they create a safe haven of support that enhances emotional resilience and motivation. This collective energy nurtures each member's journey, making the practice not merely about individual effort but also about strengthening communal bonds.

In this chapter, we explore how group mindfulness sessions can transform the experience of managing chronic pain. You'll discover the power of accountability within these groups and how shared responsibility contributes to personal growth. We'll delve into the diversity found in community settings, where each member brings unique techniques and insights to the table, enriching everyone's practice. Through stories of trust, camaraderie, and shared struggles, this chapter reveals how participation in mindfulness groups extends beyond the meditation mat to build lasting relationships that offer strength and comfort. Ultimately, you'll see how these supportive networks empower individuals to incorporate mindfulness deeply into their lives, creating pathways for both personal and community healing.

Community Mindfulness Groups

In the realm of mindfulness practice, building supportive networks through group sessions can provide incredible benefits, particularly for individuals dealing with chronic pain conditions. Being part of a community group not only encourages commitment and regular practice but also enhances motivation through shared goals and accountability. When people come together with the common purpose of practicing mindfulness, it creates an environment where everyone feels encouraged to participate and support each other's journey. This collective commitment can be a powerful motivator for maintaining a consistent practice.

One of the primary benefits of joining group mindfulness sessions is the shared sense of responsibility that arises from having mutual goals. These goals serve as compass points that guide each member, supporting their progress and holding them accountable within the group setting. When participants commit to attending regular sessions, they are more likely to engage fully and derive significant value from the experience. They feel a greater sense of duty not just to themselves but to the group as a whole, knowing that their presence contributes to the overall dynamic and energy. Giving people the opportunity to share this space allows them to make mindfulness an integral part of their lives without feeling isolated or alone in their efforts (Sutton, 2020).

Engaging with diverse group members further enriches everyone's practice by providing exposure to a variety of techniques and insights. Each person brings unique perspectives and approaches, which creates a rich tapestry of learning experiences. Participants may discover new ways to meditate that they had never considered before, or they might learn coping strategies that others have found effective in managing chronic pain. This diversity encourages open-mindedness and creativity, fostering a setting where members can learn from one another's strengths and breakthroughs.

When a group comes together with the intention of enhancing their mindfulness practice, the resulting group dynamics can elevate motivation significantly. The collective energy generated in these sessions is often greater than what any member could produce individually. It acts as a driving force that helps push personal boundaries and extends the limits of one's meditation practice. The shared energy of the group can amplify the experience, making it more rewarding and profound for all involved.

Participation in community mindfulness groups also facilitates the building of relationships that extend far beyond the meditation mat. As trust and camaraderie grow among members, so does the network of supportive connections. This sense of belonging can be especially comforting for those who suffer from chronic pain, as having a strong support system is crucial for emotional resilience. These connections foster a safe environment where individuals feel comfortable sharing their challenges and triumphs, further solidifying their bond with one another. As a result, participants are not only practicing mindfulness; they are developing meaningful relationships that offer strength and encouragement during difficult times (<i>Main Section | Community Tool Box</i>, 2025).

Importantly, the transformative nature of these group mindfulness experiences lies in their ability to nurture both individual growth and collective progress. Members witness firsthand how interconnectedness can enhance their well-being, highlighting mindfulness as a tool for both personal healing and community empowerment. By engaging with others who share similar struggles and aspirations, participants gain a deeper understanding of their own mindfulness journey and develop skills that promote long-term self-care and empathy.

For those considering joining such practices, it's essential to seek out communities with shared objectives and values that align with your own. Embracing this guideline can help ensure a fulfilling experience and contribute positively to the atmosphere of mutual respect and inspiration. It's important to remember that the relationships you build will form the foundation of your support network, reinforcing your commitment to both your practice and your peers.

Online Mindfulness Resources

In an era where technology bridges gaps and crosses boundaries, online platforms have emerged as indispensable resources for mindfulness practice. These digital spaces offer a wealth of options that cater to individuals seeking to incorporate mindfulness into their daily lives, especially those managing chronic pain. Understanding the diverse capabilities of these platforms can equip users with tools to enhance their well-being.

One of the primary benefits of online mindfulness resources is their accessibility. Virtual classes, easily accessible through various devices, allow individuals to integrate mindfulness practices seamlessly into their everyday routines. This flexibility is particularly significant for those dealing with chronic pain, as it provides the opportunity to engage in classes whether they are at home or elsewhere. The ability to tailor participation according to personal schedules without geographical limitations fosters a more consistent engagement with mindfulness practices. For instance, those who experience fluctuating pain levels can choose to attend sessions when it suits them best, thereby avoiding the strain that comes with commuting to physical locations (Roth et al., 2023).

Moreover, online platforms boast a rich variety of offerings designed to suit individual preferences. From meditation to yoga, these digital venues provide specialized content that addresses specific needs, such as chronic pain management. Through this personalized approach, practitioners can select practices that align with their unique experiences and goals. This customization is pivotal for those dealing with pain, as it allows them to explore different modalities and settle on those that yield the most relief. As one participant noted, virtual programs enable them to partake even when physical attendance isn't feasible, demonstrating the power of virtual access in pain management (Roth et al., 2023).

The capacity of online platforms to cultivate community cannot be understated. Despite the virtual nature, these platforms often foster a strong sense of belonging through forums and support groups. Individuals navigating similar challenges can connect over shared experiences, exchanging insights and offering encouragement. This collective environment not only reduces feelings of isolation but also strengthens the resolve to maintain mindfulness practices. In many cases, being part of a supportive network provides a comfort zone where individuals can express vulnerabilities and receive guidance from others on similar journeys. The camaraderie formed online mirrors traditional support systems, enriching the overall mindfulness experience by fostering interpersonal connections (Roth et al., 2023).

Continued learning represents another profound advantage of engaging with online mindfulness platforms. Regular updates to content ensure that users have access to the latest techniques and approaches. Expert talks and workshops available on these platforms serve as a valuable resource for deepening understanding and skill. They empower participants to expand their knowledge base, staying abreast of new developments in mindfulness practices. This ongoing education nurtures a culture of curiosity and growth, inviting individuals to continually refine their approaches and adapt to evolving personal needs.

Role of Peer Support in Healing

In the journey of managing chronic pain, peer relationships can serve as a crucial element in providing emotional support and facilitating healing. Individuals suffering from persistent pain often find solace in knowing that they are not alone in their struggles. Peer support offers a powerful avenue for sharing experiences, fostering understanding, and validating each other's emotions, fundamentally enhancing the emotional well-being of those involved.

One of the key aspects of peer support is its ability to reinforce feelings of understanding and shared experience. When individuals connect with others who have similar challenges, they experience emotional validation that can be profoundly comforting. This shared understanding helps in acknowledging the reality of their condition without judgment or misunderstanding, which is often encountered in other social settings (Forgeron et al., 2010). By engaging with peers who truly comprehend what living with chronic pain entails, individuals feel seen, heard, and supported. This emotional acknowledgment can alleviate feelings of isolation and decrease the psychological burden of chronic pain.

Moreover, peers play an instrumental role in motivating one another to persist in mindfulness practices. Encouragement from those who understand the intricacies of chronic pain helps maintain momentum and resolve in the face of adversity. Peers create accountability systems that encourage regular mindfulness practice, even when motivation wanes. For instance, having a partner to check in with can significantly enhance one's commitment to daily routines. This external motivation becomes invaluable during challenging times when self-discipline might falter.

Through peer support, individuals also access opportunities for mutual education and growth by exchanging techniques and insights. In these supportive settings, participants can share strategies that have been effective in managing their pain. Learning from others not only broadens an individual's repertoire of coping mechanisms but also instills a sense of empowerment through shared knowledge. These exchanges foster a learning environment where everyone benefits from the collective wisdom of the group. It transforms the management of pain into a collaborative effort rather than a solitary struggle.

Furthermore, shared experiences amongst peers build emotional resilience, creating a network of strength through stories of overcoming obstacles. Hearing about others' triumphs over similar challenges provides hope and inspiration. It reinforces the belief that progress is possible, even when faced with seemingly insurmountable hurdles. As individuals narrate their journeys, they cultivate resilience not only within themselves but also within the community they form. The act of storytelling becomes therapeutic, enabling members to process their experiences and draw strength from them (Farr et al., 2021).

A practical guideline here is to cultivate an atmosphere where encouragement and motivation are integral parts of peer interactions. This involves setting up regular meetings or check-ins, whether physically or virtually, to ensure consistent support. Group activities such as meditation sessions, workshops, or even casual gatherings focused on mindfulness practices can keep members engaged and motivated. Creating a schedule that accommodates the needs and preferences of the group helps sustain participation and reinforces a sense of commitment among peers.

Additionally, establishing a buddy system within the group acts as another layer of support. Members can pair up to provide personalized encouragement and accountability, ensuring that no one feels lost or overwhelmed in their journey towards better pain management. This system fosters deeper connections and a more personalized support structure, enhancing the overall effectiveness of the peer network.

Understanding the dynamics of peer relationships highlights their irreplaceable role in chronic pain management. These relationships not only bolster emotional support but also empower individuals to take proactive steps toward improving their quality of life. By providing a platform where lived experiences are mutually acknowledged and respected, peer networks become sanctuaries of healing and growth. They transform the experience of living with chronic pain from a solitary struggle to a shared journey, rich with understanding, motivation, and resilience.

Connecting with Mindfulness Practitioners

In the journey towards managing chronic pain through mindfulness, seeking guidance from experienced practitioners can significantly enhance one's practice. These mentors bring expertise and personalized insights that can be transformative, particularly for individuals navigating specific pain conditions. By engaging with seasoned mindfulness practitioners, learners can access tailored guidance that considers their unique circumstances. This personalized approach is crucial in ensuring that mindfulness practices not only alleviate symptoms but also provide a sustainable path for pain management.

Expert practitioners offer mentoring that involves sharing professional insights into mindfulness practices and help tailor these practices to address individual pain conditions. Such tailored guidance is vital, as it helps create a more effective and meaningful mindfulness experience by concentrating on areas needing development or adaptation. Often, chronic pain sufferers require methods that are specially adjusted to avoid exacerbating their condition while still providing mental clarity and relief. A practitioner can guide clients through this delicate balance, offering strategies that have been learned over years of dedicated practice. For instance, they might adjust the focus of meditation sessions to concentrate on breath work or body scanning techniques that are less likely to trigger discomfort yet potent enough to cultivate awareness and calm.

Moreover, committing to structured learning paths under the mentorship of professionals provides a comprehensive framework to deepen one's mindfulness journey. Professional mentors use their experience to outline progressive steps that build upon existing knowledge and adapt to the individual's pace.

This structure not only enhances commitment but also supports an individual's growth by illuminating clear pathways to follow, reducing uncertainty that often leads to discouragement. The framework acts as a roadmap, guiding practitioners through a holistic process that transforms how they manage their pain and perceive their condition over time.

Feedback and adjustment are essential aspects of mentoring relationships. They allow for continuous refinement of mindfulness approaches by identifying areas where improvement is possible and suggesting ways to achieve growth. Through regular sessions, mentors observe progress and challenges faced by individuals, offering constructive feedback that encourages adaptation and experimentation within practice. This iterative process helps refine techniques, such as focusing attention or cultivating compassion, so they become more effective and fit seamlessly into daily routines. Receiving ongoing input ensures that practices remain dynamic and relevant, preventing stagnation and encouraging constant evolution of the practice.

Establishing connections with mindfulness practitioners inherently builds motivation and fosters commitment. These relationships create a supportive environment where trust is nurtured and maintained over time. Knowing that there is someone knowledgeable to turn to when difficulties arise can greatly enhance a practitioner's motivation to continue despite setbacks. This network of support reassures individuals that they are not alone in their journey, which can be empowering and motivating. Practitioners serve as allies who hold space for exploration, helping to sustain momentum through encouragement and shared wisdom.

A meaningful mentor-mentee relationship is built upon trust and open dialogue. As trust deepens, mentees are more likely to express concerns and questions, leading to richer discussions and more profound insights. This ongoing interaction can instill a sense of accountability, as mentees feel encouraged to stay consistent with their practice out of respect for their mentor and their own progress. The reciprocal nature of support in these relationships nourishes both parties, with practitioners often finding renewed inspiration in the progress and dedication of those they mentor.

For individuals dealing with chronic pain, such guided mindfulness practice can be life-changing. By working closely with practitioners who understand the complexities of their condition and can provide expert advice, they are equipped to embrace mindfulness as a viable strategy for pain management. This holistic approach not only addresses physical discomfort but also enriches emotional well-being, allowing individuals to lead more fulfilled lives.

Value of Shared Experiences

Sharing personal journeys in mindfulness communities can significantly enhance collective growth. One of the most powerful methods to achieve this is through storytelling as a form of healing. Within these communities, sharing personal experiences doesn't just recount individual tales; it weaves a tapestry of shared understanding and empathy. When individuals open up about their own challenges and triumphs, it fosters a therapeutic environment where everyone feels connected. In doing so, they provide a source of inspiration for others facing similar struggles, offering new perspectives and hope.

The act of storytelling within these settings serves as a bridge, uniting diverse experiences and backgrounds. It allows members to see beyond their own circumstances and appreciate the resilience in others, reinforcing the notion that no one is alone on this journey. Personal narratives have the ability to transcend cultural and social boundaries, creating a sense of unity and shared purpose among participants. This connection is vital for those managing chronic pain, as it reminds them they are part of a supportive network that understands their journey intimately.

Another benefit of sharing stories in mindfulness communities is the emergence of collective wisdom through group discussions. These conversations, enriched by diverse experiences, often yield insights that might be difficult to reach individually. Group interactions allow members to bounce ideas off each other, leading to profound realizations and strategies for coping with stress and pain. Hearing different viewpoints expands one's own perspective, encouraging a more holistic approach to mindfulness practices. For instance, someone may discover a technique they'd never considered but find surprisingly effective, thanks to a member's contribution.

Additionally, creating a safe space within these communities is paramount for fostering vulnerability and open expression of emotions. This environment not only encourages individuals to share their narratives but also provides reassurance that their feelings will be met with understanding and respect. Establishing such trust is crucial, especially for people dealing with chronic pain who may feel isolated or misunderstood in other aspects of their lives. Guidelines for creating a safe space include setting clear boundaries for confidentiality and encouraging active listening without judgment. By cultivating this atmosphere, participants can express their emotions freely, knowing that they are supported and valued.

A safe space also nurtures the courage to be vulnerable, which is essential in forging deeper connections. When individuals witness others expressing their truths without fear of rejection, it creates a ripple effect, emboldening everyone to participate more fully. Vulnerability becomes a shared experience that strengthens the group's overall cohesion. Over time, this openness leads to stronger emotional bonds, enabling members to support each other on a deeper level, both during and outside formal sessions.

Strengthening community bonds through shared experiences is another critical aspect of building robust support networks. The shared experiences within mindfulness groups create memories and touchpoints that continually reinforce the network's strength. As members engage in group activities, whether it's meditation sessions, retreats, or casual gatherings, they build a repository of positive shared experiences. These moments contribute to a sense of belonging and solidarity, vital ingredients in any supportive community.

The cumulative effect of these shared experiences contributes to the resilience of the group. Knowing that others have faced and overcome similar challenges adds a layer of communal strength. It awakens a spirit of camaraderie that can be transformative for individuals feeling overwhelmed by their circumstances. Chronic pain sufferers can find solace and empowerment in this collective strength, which bolsters their capacity to cope and thrive despite ongoing challenges.

Moreover, engaging in shared practices solidifies the community's commitment to each other's well-being. Activities such as group meditations or mindful walks serve not only to enhance individual mindfulness practices but also to cement interpersonal relationships. Through these interactions, members reinforce their dedication to maintaining a nurturing environment where everyone's contributions are valued. This mutual investment supports the long-term sustainability of the community, ensuring it remains a vibrant, living entity capable of adapting and evolving with its members' needs.

Ultimately, the collective growth achieved through sharing personal journeys within mindfulness communities underscores the power of human connection in healing. By weaving together storytelling, collective wisdom, safe spaces, and strengthened bonds, these communities become more than just support networks; they transform into life-affirming ecosystems that inspire and elevate every participant. Such environments not only aid in managing chronic pain but also enhance the overall quality of participants' lives, providing them with tools and connections that resonate far beyond their mindfulness practice.

Concluding Thoughts

In this chapter, we've explored the profound impact of building supportive networks for mindfulness practice, especially valuable for those dealing with chronic pain. By joining community mindfulness groups, individuals can find motivation and a sense of accountability that encourages regular practice. The presence of like-minded peers strengthens commitment and provides a deeper understanding of mindfulness through collective experience. This shared journey not only nurtures personal growth but also weaves a fabric of strong relationships, offering emotional resilience during tough times. Through diverse interactions, members gain insights into new techniques and coping strategies, enriching their mindfulness repertoire.

As we reflect on the value of these connections, it's evident how essential they are in transforming mindfulness into a cornerstone of daily life. The communal aspect fosters a reassuring environment where encouragement flourishes, making the path to healing less solitary. These networks become sanctuaries of empathy and support, empowering individuals to address both their physical discomfort and emotional well-being. As you continue your journey, consider integrating into communities that resonate with your goals and values, nurturing your practice and reinforcing the bonds you build within them.

Reference List

Author, S. development. (2023, May 18). *Unearthing the Secret to Amplified Personal Growth: Collective Mindfulness*. Medium. https://medium.com/@yacuncao2/unearthing-the-secret-to-amplified-personal-growth-collective-mindfulness-61595f0779bc

Forgeron, P. A., King, S., Stinson, J. N., McGrath, P. J., MacDonald, A. J., & Chambers, C. T. (2010). *Social functioning and peer relationships in children and adolescents with chronic pain: A systematic review.* Pain Research & Management; Pulsus Group Inc. https://doi.org/10.1155/2010/820407

Farr, M., Brant, H., Patel, R., Linton, M.-J., Ambler, N., Vyas, S., Wedge, H., Watkins, S., & Horwood, J. (2021, June 28). *Experiences of Patient-Led Chronic Pain Peer Support Groups After Pain Management Programs: A Qualitative Study.* Pain Medicine. https://doi.org/10.1093/pm/pnab189

How to create a supportive environment for residents with chronic pain. (2025). Downersgrovehc.com. https://www.downersgrovehc.com/blog/how-to-create-a-supportive-environment-for-residents-with-chronic-pain?372b7fa3_page=3

Main Section | Community Tool Box. (2025). Ku.edu. http://ctb.ku.edu/en/table-of-contents/spirituality-and-community-building/mindfulness-community-building/main

Mindfulness Mentoring | The Mindfulness Network. (2020, July 2). The Mindfulness Network | Serving the Community through Mindfulness-Based Supervision, Retreats and Training Courses. http://home.mindfulness-network.org/practice-mindfulness/mindfulness-mentoring/

Meditative Journey: Storytelling in Guided Meditation. (2023). Themindorchestra.com. https://www.themindorchestra.com/blog/meditative-guided-meditation-storytelling

New. (2021). *Deep Mindfulness*. Deep Mindfulness. https://deepmindfulness.io/mentorship

Roth, I., Tiedt, M., Miller, V., Barnhill, J., Chilcoat, A., Gardiner, P., Faurot, K., Karvelas, K., Busby, K., Gaylord, S., & Leeman, J. (2023, September 27). *Integrative medical group visits for patients with chronic pain: results of a pilot single-site hybrid implementation-effectiveness feasibility study*. Frontiers in Pain Research. https://doi.org/10.3389/fpain.2023.1147588

Sutton, J. (2020, July 24). *Practicing Mindfulness in Groups: 9 Activities and Exercises*. PositivePsychology.com. https://positivepsychology.com/group-mindfulness-activities/

CHAPTER 13

Overcoming Obstacles to Mindfulness

Overcoming obstacles to mindfulness can be particularly challenging for those managing chronic pain, as each day brings its own set of battles. The practice of mindfulness offers a refuge amidst these challenges, providing a path toward inner peace and resilience. Yet, many individuals find themselves struggling to sustain this practice due to the various hurdles that arise along the journey. These barriers may seem insurmountable at times, but recognizing them is the first step toward effective management. Identifying and understanding what impedes one's progress lays the groundwork for cultivating a more meaningful and consistent mindfulness practice.

In this chapter, we delve into some of the most common obstacles faced by individuals on their mindfulness journey. We explore how the fast-paced demands of modern life often leave little time for introspection and how distractions, both external and internal, constantly pull attention away from the present moment. Addressing self-doubt is also crucial, as these feelings can undermine one's confidence in their ability to master mindfulness techniques. Physical discomfort presents another significant challenge, particularly for those dealing with chronic pain, necessitating adaptive strategies. By understanding these barriers and discovering personalized solutions, readers will find practical advice to support their ongoing commitment to mindfulness.

Identifying Common Obstacles

In the journey towards mindfulness, recognizing and understanding the barriers that may impede your progress is essential for cultivating a sustainable practice. Let's explore some common obstacles and potential ways to overcome them.

Lack of Time

One of the most frequently cited hurdles in practicing mindfulness is the lack of time. In today's fast-paced world, our schedules are crammed with countless responsibilities, leaving little room for introspection or meditative practices. However, integrating mindfulness into daily routines is indeed possible and can be profoundly beneficial. Consider starting small by setting aside short, intentional intervals throughout the day dedicated to mindfulness. This could be as simple as five minutes of deep breathing during your lunch break, observing your surroundings on your commute, or even mindful eating at dinner (Change, 2021). The key is to make mindfulness a seamless part of your daily schedule, thus fostering consistent practice without overwhelming yourself.

Identifying Distractions

Distractions abound in our modern lives, often pulling us away from being present in the moment. By identifying specific distractions, you can employ techniques that help enhance your focus during mindfulness exercises. Consider keeping a distraction journal where you note down recurrent interruptions and analyze their patterns. Are these distractions external, like noise or digital notifications, or internal, such as wandering thoughts about tasks yet to be completed? Once identified, tailor solutions to these distractions: create a quiet space free from gadgets when practicing, or use mindfulness apps designed to lead your focus gently back to the present moment despite occasional disruptions. Recognizing these distractions allows individuals to take proactive steps toward creating an environment conducive to mindfulness (Schuman-Olivier et al., 2020).

Overcoming Self-Doubt

Self-doubt can significantly hinder one's mindfulness journey, evoking feelings that one isn't making progress or is doing the practice 'incorrectly.' Acknowledging these feelings, however, is the first step towards dispelling them. Celebrate the small victories—whether it's taking time out for a single mindful breath or resisting the urge to judge your experience harshly. These acknowledgments help build confidence and reinforce the understanding that mindfulness is a journey, not a destination. It's vital to remember that every moment of presence counts and contributes to strengthening your overall practice.

Physical Discomfort

Finally, physical discomfort poses a substantial challenge, especially for individuals managing chronic pain conditions. Traditional mindfulness practices like sitting meditation might exacerbate physical discomfort, leading to frustration. Adaptation becomes key in this context. Modify your posture or explore different types of mindfulness exercises that accommodate your body's needs. Mindful walking, gentle yoga, or body scans can serve as alternatives that allow for continued practice despite physical limitations. Moreover, this adaptation not only promotes persistence but also provides positive feedback on pain management, empowering individuals to understand and mitigate their discomfort through mindful awareness (Change, 2021).

Strategies for Maintaining Motivation

In the journey of mindfulness, many individuals encounter hurdles that challenge their resolve. However, by implementing strategic approaches, one can maintain consistent motivation and dedication to this transformative practice. To begin with, clearly defining personal intentions serves as a cornerstone for sustaining mindfulness. Intentions act like the compass guiding each individual's unique path, offering direction and meaning. By setting clear goals such as reducing stress or cultivating self-awareness, practitioners create a tangible purpose. This sense of purpose not only drives ongoing commitment but also acts as an anchor during moments when motivation wanes. Setting these intentions involves reflection and honesty about what you genuinely seek from your practice.

One effective strategy is to start each day by revisiting these intentions. This simple morning routine helps align actions with desires, fostering consistency. An intention might be something as simple as embracing patience or practicing gratitude. The key is maintaining clarity, which strengthens the connection between thought and action, making it easier to stick to mindful living (Pal et al., 2018). Consistency in reaffirming intentions imbues daily actions with significance, ensuring that the practice of mindfulness is consciously integrated into life.

Tracking progress further augments motivation. Life can get overwhelming, and sometimes the slow pace of change tempers enthusiasm. Journaling emerges as a powerful tool here, allowing practitioners to document their experiences, thoughts, and feelings. A journal not only records progress but also provides a space for reflective insight. Writing down occurrences or emotional shifts can illuminate subtle yet significant changes over time, validating one's efforts. Visual indicators, like charts or mood boards, can serve as engaging ways to track growth, making achievements more palpable. This visual feedback loop reinforces commitment as individuals witness tangible evidence of their journey's impact.

Another method to sustain motivation is joining a community of like-minded individuals. Engaging with groups—whether online or in person—creates accountability and shared experience. Community support offers a network of encouragement, where members can exchange insights, share challenges, and celebrate milestones. Such environments nurture empathy and understanding, enhancing the richness of the mindfulness journey. While the solitude of mindfulness is its charm, human connection brings added dimensions of growth. Dialogue within these communities often sparks inspiration and renews vigor to persevere through difficulties (Madeson, 2022).

Variety is equally crucial in combating monotony, which can stifle engagement. Mixing different mindfulness practices is a way to avoid falling into a routine that feels stale. Exploring various techniques—such as walking meditation, body scans, or loving-kindness exercises—prevents predictability from dampening enthusiasm. Each practice offers distinct benefits and perspectives, enriching the overall experience. By experimenting, practitioners discover which methods resonate most deeply, tailoring mindfulness to fit evolving needs and interests. This variety ensures that practice remains fresh and stimulating, prompting sustained involvement (Pal et al., 2018).

Moreover, acknowledging the flexibility in mixing practices allows for adaptability. On days when sitting for extended periods seems daunting, shorter, more dynamic practices can retain attention and interest. The freedom to choose among a range of activities fosters a sense of autonomy, vital for long-term commitment. By creating a repertoire of practices, individuals position themselves to respond dynamically to their current state of mind or environment, thus maintaining engagement.

Finally, while motivation ebbs and flows naturally, celebrating small achievements within the journey plays a pivotal role in sustaining effort. Each step taken, no matter how incremental, signifies progress, reinforcing perseverance. Acknowledging these victories, either through personal reflection or within a community, bolsters confidence and affirms the value of continued practice. This positive reinforcement cultivates resilience, empowering individuals to weather challenges and continue on their path with renewed determination.

Dealing with Setbacks

In the pursuit of mindfulness, setbacks are simply part of the journey. They are not indicative of failure but rather milestones that signal growth and learning. Embracing this truth is essential to maintaining motivation and progress in mindfulness practices. Recognizing setbacks as a normal occurrence can alleviate feelings of inadequacy. This perspective fosters a more forgiving and realistic approach, enabling practitioners to engage with their challenges constructively. As individuals acknowledge setbacks as natural, they become integral to the mastery of mindfulness, facilitating long-term growth and resilience.

An important strategy for managing these inevitable disruptions involves reflection—a thoughtful process that encourages adaptation and personalization of mindfulness practices. By examining moments where obstacles arise, practitioners gain insights into patterns or triggers that may need addressing. For example, if stress often interrupts meditation sessions, one might explore strategies to establish a more conducive environment or time for practice. Reflection provides an opportunity to evaluate what works and what doesn't, allowing mindfulness routines to evolve naturally over time. This adaptability ensures that practices remain sustainable and effective, even amidst changing circumstances. Applying these reflections meaningfully can reinforce future endeavors and bolster one's commitment to mindfulness.

Guidance on reflecting effectively includes taking deliberate pauses to consider specific setbacks and asking critical questions that probe deeper understanding: What factors contributed to this interruption? How did it affect my emotional state? What could be adjusted or tried differently next time? These inquiries help transform potential frustrations into learning experiences, supporting a constructive cycle of improvement and self-awareness.

Another pivotal element in overcoming setbacks is the role of support systems. Engaging with communities, whether through formal groups or informal networks, offers vital connection and encouragement during challenging times. Support from others provides a platform for shared experiences, enabling individuals to draw inspiration and reassurance from those who have faced similar hurdles. Whether through online forums, local meet-ups, or mindfulness classes, the sense of unity can rekindle motivation and provide much-needed empathy when personal resolve wavers. Friends, mentors, or fellow practitioners act as sounding boards, offering fresh perspectives and emotional sustenance.

Furthermore, practicing self-compassion is a fundamental aspect of maintaining a positive outlook on one's mindfulness journey. Often, individuals experiencing setbacks may succumb to harsh self-criticism, undermining the essence of mindfulness itself. Instead, approaching oneself with kindness and understanding transforms setbacks into opportunities for nurturing growth. Adopting a gentle internal dialogue reminds practitioners that mistakes are human and that learning is valuable regardless of any missteps along the way.

For instance, when missing a meditation session, rather than dwelling on disappointment, one might remind themselves that tomorrow is another opportunity. Acknowledging personal efforts, however small, reinforces a compassionate mindset— one rooted in acceptance and patience. In embracing self-compassion, practitioners create a safe space within themselves to explore mindfulness without fear of judgment, ultimately promoting a healthier and more effective practice.

To illustrate, consider implementing simple affirmations that encourage a supportive inner voice, such as "I am learning at my own pace" or "This is part of my journey." Such affirmations serve as gentle reminders that success lies not in perfection but in persistent effort and engagement.

Finally, integrating these strategies holistically paves the way for a more resilient mindfulness journey, helping individuals to manage setbacks gracefully and with renewed purpose. Setbacks do not signify defeat; instead, they offer unique opportunities for introspection, community involvement, and self-kindness. By understanding and accepting these principles, practitioners can navigate their challenges confidently, ensuring a sustainable path toward mindfulness that respects the inevitable ebbs and flows of life.

Managing Time Effectively

Incorporating mindfulness into a busy life can be challenging but immensely rewarding. Prioritizing mindfulness as an essential daily activity ensures that it becomes a natural part of your routine rather than an add-on. To do this, one might need to reconsider their current daily schedule and identify opportunities where mindfulness can be seamlessly integrated. This could start with the simple act of setting aside a few minutes each morning for a brief meditation or reflection session, providing a calm and focused start to the day.

For those pressed for time, emphasizing short practices is crucial. It's a common misconception that effective mindfulness requires extended periods of meditation. In reality, even a few minutes of mindful breathing or observation can significantly impact one's mental well-being. For instance, during moments of waiting—whether in a queue or at traffic lights—one can practice mindful breathing. This not only uses time efficiently but also demonstrates the quality-over-quantity principle that is central to mindfulness (Self-Care for the Busy Professional: Quick and Effective Strategies - Routine & Habit Tracker App Tips: Better Life with Routinery, 2024).

Limiting screen time can also play a pivotal role in creating space for mindfulness. Many individuals find themselves absorbed by their devices, whether it's scrolling through social media or checking emails late into the night. Allocating specific times to check devices helps reduce digital fatigue. Instead of spending breaks on screens, consider using these intervals for short mindfulness exercises, such as deep breathing or body scans. By creating tech-free zones at home where no devices are allowed, you can foster an environment more conducive to mindfulness practice. This frees up valuable time and mental space for engaging in mindful activities and reduces the overwhelm often associated with constant connectivity (for, 2024).

Another strategy involves establishing consistent routines which provide structure, making it easier to integrate mindfulness into everyday habits. Regularity in practice offers predictability and comfort, fostering a stable mental state necessary for mindfulness. For example, coupling mindfulness with daily activities—such as mindful eating during meals or practicing gratitude before bedtime—can solidify its place in your routine. Having set times for these practices transforms them from tasks into ingrained habits that promote sustained mindfulness over time.

Using technology wisely can further aid these efforts. There are numerous apps designed to send reminders or guide users through brief meditation sessions, enabling even the busiest individuals to access mindfulness tools when they need them most. Exploring different app features can help find what best fits personal schedules and preferences, ensuring that mindfulness remains an accessible and tailored experience.

Additionally, prioritizing mindfulness requires acknowledging it as vital for overall well-being. Understanding its benefits helps cultivate intrinsic motivation to practice regularly. Mindfulness is known to enhance focus, reduce stress, and improve emotional health, offering a compelling reason to make it a priority. Recognizing these advantages encourages individuals to keep mindfulness at the forefront of their daily agendas.

To truly embed mindfulness into one's lifestyle, flexibility is key. Busy lives are unpredictable, so being adaptable ensures that practice can continue despite changing circumstances. If a planned meditation session is missed due to an unforeseen commitment, finding another moment—even if just a minute or two—to breathe deeply and refocus can still uphold the practice's essence. Such adaptability reinforces a commitment to mindfulness without inducing guilt or pressure.

Lastly, sharing the journey with others can offer additional support and encouragement. Discussing experiences with friends, family, or mindfulness communities can provide fresh insights and mutual motivation, enhancing personal practice while fostering a sense of belonging. These shared experiences underline the universal challenges of maintaining mindfulness amidst life's demands, reminding practitioners they are not alone in their endeavors.

Creating a Supportive Environment

Creating an environment conducive to mindfulness practice is a transformative step for individuals seeking to manage chronic pain through alternative methods. By designing spaces with intention, one can foster a sense of peace and focus necessary for effective mindfulness. A designated mindfulness space does wonders in facilitating the transition into a mindful state consistently. Much like a sanctuary, this space becomes a refuge from the chaos of the outside world, allowing the mind and body to settle. It doesn't have to be elaborate—just a quiet corner with a comfortable cushion or chair, perhaps near a window with natural light, can serve as your personal retreat. The simplicity of this setup helps signal to the mind that it's time to engage in mindfulness, creating a habitual mental response over time.

Minimizing clutter within this space further enhances mental clarity and focus during mindfulness sessions. Clutter not only distracts visually but also mentally, as it often represents unfinished tasks or decisions yet to be made. Clearing out unnecessary items creates a clean slate, inviting calmness and tranquility. This minimalistic approach fosters an environment where attention can be focused inward without external distractions pulling one's thoughts away. As the saying goes, a tidy space makes for a tidy mind, which is especially crucial when one aims to delve deep into mindfulness practice.

Incorporating visual reminders throughout spaces can act as gentle prompts for regular mindfulness breaks. Consider placing small cues around the home or workspace, such as inspirational quotes, serene images, or objects that hold personal significance. These elements serve as momentary pauses, encouraging brief return trips to a state of mindfulness even amidst the busyness of daily life. This practice aligns well with the notion of becoming more present in the current moment, as these cues draw our attention back to what is happening now, rather than what has passed or may come. They act as anchors, supporting the journey toward greater awareness and emotional regulation.

Inviting positive influences from supportive peers nurtures a commitment to mindfulness practices by providing encouragement and a sense of community. Engaging with others who share similar goals offers accountability and shared experiences, fostering motivation to remain dedicated to the practice. This sense of belonging can be integral, especially when exploring new habits or paradigms in managing chronic pain. Having a network of like-minded individuals provides opportunities for discussion, learning, and even participating in group mindfulness activities, enriching the experience and reinforcing its importance in one's life.

Designing a supportive environment for mindfulness involves thoughtful consideration of physical and social elements that contribute to a nurturing atmosphere. Designating a specific mindfulness space sets the stage for consistent practice, while minimizing clutter enhances the potential for mental clarity. Visual reminders serve as beacons guiding one back to mindfulness throughout the day. Finally, surrounding oneself with positive influences ensures that the practice is sustained through community support and shared encouragement.

It is essential to recognize that creating such an environment requires an understanding of personal needs and preferences. Each person's definition of tranquility and focus may differ, and thus, each mindfulness space should be uniquely tailored. Whether it involves adding soft lighting, calming scents, or incorporating nature-inspired decor, the idea is to construct a haven that resonates personally and supports the mindfulness journey.

With these elements in place, not only does one create a conducive setting for mindfulness, but they also foster a lifestyle change that aligns with broader life goals. The act of intentionally designing such a space signifies a commitment to personal growth and self-care, a powerful statement in itself. Over time, this environment will naturally encourage more profound engagement in mindfulness practices, promoting greater awareness and management of pain symptoms.

Moreover, these strategies are accessible to everyone, regardless of space or budget constraints. Creativity and intentionality are key, allowing anyone to transform existing environments into spaces that nurture mindfulness. Whether a full room dedicated to practice or merely a corner with a few select items, the impact on one's mindfulness journey can be significant.

Concluding Thoughts

Throughout this chapter, we've explored the various challenges in maintaining a mindfulness practice, particularly for those managing chronic pain. Recognizing obstacles like time constraints, distractions, self-doubt, and physical discomfort is the first step toward addressing them effectively. By acknowledging these barriers, individuals can begin to integrate mindfulness into their daily lives more seamlessly. Whether it's carving out brief moments for mindfulness amid busy schedules or adapting practices to accommodate physical limitations, every effort counts. The journey may not always be straightforward, but patience and persistence are central to cultivating a sustainable mindfulness routine.

Additionally, building a supportive environment plays a crucial role in encouraging continued practice. Creating dedicated spaces free from clutter and filled with calming elements can enhance focus and tranquility. Engaging with communities that share similar goals also offers valuable support, allowing individuals to draw on collective wisdom and encouragement. This shared journey reinforces the idea that you're not alone in navigating life's complexities. As you continue exploring mindfulness, remember that each small step forward contributes to your growth and resilience, helping you manage pain with greater awareness and compassion.

Reference List

Bansal, M. (2020, January 30). *Encouraging Mindfulness Through Design - Mihika Bansal - Medium*. Medium. https://mihikabansal.medium.com/encouraging-mindfulness-through-design-7e7465235830

Change, I. (2021, August 24). *How to Overcome Obstacles to Mindfulness.* Intelligent Change. https://www.intelligentchange.com/blogs/read/how-to-overcome-obstacles-to-mindfulness?srsltid=AfmBOorFIOmw9KN_Umow4gbnn-l1OMsfC5q6NR6QG07oJCZefLFHyIzN

Five Healthy Coping Skills For Facing Setbacks | BetterHelp. (n.d.). Www.betterhelp.com. https://www.betterhelp.com/advice/mindfulness/five-healthy-coping-skills-for-facing-setbacks/

Grant. (2022, March 29). *Dr. Daya Grant*. Dr. Daya Grant. https://www.dayagrant.com/blog/a-mindful-strategy-for-facing-setbacks

Madeson, M. (2022, October 27). *Mindfulness in counseling: 8 best techniques & interventions*. PositivePsychology.com. https://positivepsychology.com/mindfulness-in-counseling/

Pal, P., Hauck, C., Goldstein, E., Bobinet, K., & Bradley, C. (2018, December 13). *5 simple mindfulness practices for daily life*. Mindful. https://www.mindful.org/take-a-mindful-moment-5-simple-practices-for-daily-life/

Schuman-Olivier, Z., Trombka, M., Lovas, D. A., Brewer, J. A., Vago, D. R., Gawande, R., Dunne, J. P., Lazar, S. W., Loucks, E. B., & Fulwiler, C. (2020). *Mindfulness and behavior change*. Harvard Review of Psychiatry. https://doi.org/10.1097/HRP.0000000000000277

Self-Care for the Busy Professional: Quick and Effective Strategies - Routine & Habit Tracker App Tips: Better Life with Routinery. (2024, February 15). Routinery.app. https://routinery.app/blog/selfcare-for-the-busy-professional-quick-and-effective-strategies-16183

Team, T. (2025, February 13). *How Mindfulness Influences your Design Thinking*. Timely.com; Timely Blog. https://www.timely.com/blog/how-mindfulness-influences-your-design-thinking

for, S. (2024, August 26). *7 Self-Care Strategies for Busy Professionals*. Little Rock Center. https://rhlittlerock.com/blog/7-self-care-strategies-for-busy-professionals

CHAPTER 14

Cultural Perspectives on Pain and Healing

Cultural perspectives on pain and healing offer a fascinating lens through which to view human experiences across different societies. These perspectives shape how individuals perceive, manage, and heal from pain, intertwining deeply with spiritual beliefs, values, and social norms. The chapter delves into this complex interplay, shedding light on the rich diversity of viewpoints that exist in our global tapestry. By examining how various cultures approach the concepts of discomfort and recovery, we can broaden our understanding and appreciation for the multitude of methods people use to seek relief and achieve balance.

This chapter explores both Eastern and Western perspectives on pain and healing, highlighting their unique approaches as well as commonalities. You'll find insights into traditional Eastern philosophies, such as those from China and India, which emphasize holistic practices like acupuncture and Ayurveda. Meanwhile, Western medical views reveal an evolution towards integrative approaches that merge biomedical models with psychological therapies, including mindfulness-based interventions. Additionally, the text will introduce cross-cultural mindfulness practices that serve as collective bridges to wellness, and address the importance of cultural sensitivity in healthcare settings. By traveling through these multifaceted cultural viewpoints, readers are invited to discover new dimensions of managing pain beyond conventional boundaries, enriching their healing journey with wisdom drawn from diverse traditions.

Traditional Eastern Perspectives

Eastern philosophies offer rich insights into the complex dynamics of pain and healing, emphasizing an integrated approach that considers the body, mind, and spirit as a unified whole. Central to many of these Eastern traditions is the concept of Qi, which refers to vital energy flow within the body. Imbalances or blockages in Qi are believed to result in physical discomfort and illness. Practices such as acupuncture, a key component of Traditional Chinese Medicine, are employed to restore this balance. By inserting fine needles into specific points on the body, acupuncture seeks to unblock Qi pathways, promoting the body's natural healing processes. This practice not only aims to alleviate immediate pain but also encourages long-term wellness by addressing underlying energetic imbalances (Elendu, 2024).

In India, Ayurveda presents a complementary yet distinct perspective on health and healing. This ancient system emphasizes the balance of body, mind, and spirit through individualized approaches, including dietary choices and yoga practices. Ayurvedic principles focus on maintaining harmony among the three doshas—Vata, Pitta, and Kapha—believed to govern bodily functions and mental states. For individuals experiencing chronic pain, Ayurveda recommends personalized dietary regimens and lifestyle adjustments designed to restore balance and promote healing from within. Yoga, a significant element of Ayurvedic practice, facilitates physical alignment and mental clarity, providing tools for individuals to manage pain through enhanced self-awareness and relaxation techniques (Elendu, 2024).

Mindfulness and meditation are integral components across various Eastern philosophies, offering profound insights into managing and understanding chronic pain. These practices emphasize acceptance and awareness, encouraging individuals to observe their pain without judgment or resistance. By cultivating mindfulness, people learn to navigate their discomfort with compassion rather than fear, reducing anxiety and altering their perception of pain. Meditation techniques help shift focus from the pain itself to a more holistic understanding of one's experience, fostering resilience and enhancing emotional regulation. Through consistent practice, mindfulness and meditation can significantly impact how individuals cope with chronic pain, transforming their relationship with it from one of fear to acceptance (*Ikigai Transfromations- Live on Purpose*, 2024).

Community support plays a crucial role in amplifying the benefits of mindfulness and meditation. Collective rituals and shared experiences provide individuals with a sense of belonging and reinforce the healing power of mindfulness. In many Eastern traditions, group meditation sessions or community gatherings are common, offering participants a supportive environment to explore their emotions and share their journeys. These communal settings foster connection and empathy, helping individuals realize they are not alone in their struggles. By participating in these collective activities, people strengthen their mindfulness practice, receiving encouragement and inspiration from others on similar paths. Community engagement thus enhances personal healing and contributes to the overall well-being of the group, highlighting the transformative potential of shared human experiences (*Ikigai Transfromations- Live on Purpose*, 2024).

Western Medical Viewpoints

In Western medical approaches, the treatment of pain is often viewed through the lens of the biomedical model. This perspective considers pain as a purely physical symptom resulting from a detectable abnormality in the body. Consequently, treatments traditionally focus on physical interventions such as medication or surgery to alleviate symptoms. For instance, pain management might include prescribing analgesics or conducting surgical procedures aimed at correcting physical issues like herniated discs or joint problems.

However, over time, practitioners have recognized that pain is not solely a physiological experience but also encompasses psychological and social dimensions. Hence, Cognitive Behavioral Therapy (CBT) has emerged to address these aspects by helping individuals modify unhelpful cognitive patterns. CBT provides tools to manage pain by changing thought processes related to discomfort, thus complementing traditional methods with mindfulness practices. In fact, mindfulness techniques are integrated within CBT frameworks to promote awareness and acceptance of sensations without judgment (Hofmann & Gómez, 2018).

Research has increasingly validated mindfulness as an effective tool in managing pain, extending beyond conventional medical treatments. Mindfulness-based interventions (MBIs), such as Mindfulness-Based Stress Reduction (MBSR) and

Mindfulness-Based Cognitive Therapy (MBCT), significantly reduce anxiety and depression, which can exacerbate perceptions of pain. Studies show that MBIs consistently outperform non-evidence-based treatments and perform comparably to established therapies like CBT. By encouraging present-moment awareness, mindfulness helps individuals become less reactive to pain, fostering a more reflective state that aids in reducing stress and enhancing well-being (Hofmann & Gómez, 2018).

Mindfulness is beneficial for its ability to enhance patient-centered care, which emphasizes the active involvement of patients in their healing journey. Unlike traditional models where individuals may feel passive in their treatment, patient-centered care empowers them to become active participants. This approach encourages ongoing dialogue between healthcare providers and patients, ensuring treatments align with personal values and preferences. When patients engage actively in their care, they report a greater sense of control and satisfaction, which is especially vital in chronic pain management.

To fully integrate mindfulness with Western medical treatments, it requires addressing several components and guidelines. While mindfulness meditation, yoga, and tai chi are pivotal, there's an emphasis on creating intentional patient-care plans tailored to individual needs. Ensuring a holistic, person-centered approach involves understanding patients' beliefs and responding empathetically to their experiences of pain. Healthcare professionals must cultivate a compassionate and supportive environment where mindfulness practices are accessible and augment traditional care.

The incorporation of mindfulness into Western medicine is also supported by robust evidence. Trials comparing MBSR and MBCT to control conditions indicate effectiveness across diverse populations, showing improvements in various disorders, including chronic pain, stress, and emotional distress. As mental health nurses and other frontline practitioners adopt this more holistic approach, they find greater capacity to assess, intervene, and support individuals throughout their health journeys. The increased emphasis on mindfulness in care aligns with principles of compassion, empathy, and therapeutic relationships founded on presence and acceptance (AlSubaie et al., 2024).

Patient-centered care further enhances these benefits by validating the patient's voice in their own healing. When mindfulness becomes part of routine practice, patients often develop coping skills that improve both psychological resilience and physiological outcomes. They learn to appreciate the mind-body connection, recognizing how thoughts and emotions can influence their perception of pain. By fostering mindful awareness, individuals gain insight into their experiences, leading to empowerment and informed choices about their healing path.

For those seeking alternative methods to manage chronic pain, integrating mindfulness with traditional medical approaches offers several advantages. Not only does it provide a comprehensive framework that addresses physical, mental, and emotional components of pain, but it also respects each individual's unique journey. Through patient-centered care models and ongoing research, the harmonization of mindfulness in Western medicine continues to evolve, promising better outcomes and quality of life for those living with chronic pain.

Cross-Cultural Mindfulness Practices

In many cultures, mindfulness practices have been recognized as powerful tools for managing pain and promoting healing. Around the globe, these practices reflect a rich tapestry of cultural diversity, which offers valuable methods to broaden our understanding and approaches to pain reduction.

Firstly, it's important to recognize how cultural variability in mindfulness practices can contribute uniquely to pain management. Each culture brings its own perspective, often shaped by historical experiences and social contexts. In some Asian traditions, mindfulness is deeply rooted in spiritual practice and daily routine. The Buddhist concept of mindfulness, or 'sati', emphasizes awareness and acceptance of the present moment, which has been shown to reduce emotional suffering and physical pain (Schuman-Olivier et al., 2020). By integrating such techniques into modern wellness practices, individuals can experience a greater sense of control and comfort over chronic pain conditions.

Indigenous traditions around the world also emphasize daily rituals that foster community cohesion and provide individuals with a sense of purpose. These rituals often incorporate elements of mindfulness, focusing on communal activities that encourage participants to be present and engaged. In Native American cultures, for instance, ceremonial practices such as sweat lodges or drumming circles are not only spiritual but also therapeutic, offering a holistic approach to health and wellbeing. Such rituals support both physical healing and psychological resilience by grounding individuals in their communities and connecting them to ancestral wisdom. The active engagement in these shared experiences can act as a buffer against the isolating effects of chronic pain, fostering a sense of belonging and mutual support.

Among the diverse array of mindfulness techniques, walking meditation stands out as a particularly accessible and enriching practice. This form of meditation, prevalent in various cultures, involves intentional focus on the movement and sensations of walking. It's an effective method for cultivating mindfulness because it combines physical activity with meditative awareness. Walking meditation helps individuals connect with their bodies, providing a gentle way to alleviate pain by encouraging movement without strain. Moreover, it promotes mental clarity and emotional calmness, helping to diffuse stress and anxiety, which can exacerbate pain symptoms (Kriakous et al., 2021).

For those interested in incorporating walking meditation into their routine, begin by selecting a quiet, pleasant environment where you can walk without interruptions. Walk at a slow pace, paying attention to each step, the sensation of your feet touching the ground, and the rhythm of your breathing. If your mind wanders, gently bring your attention back to these sensations. Start with short sessions and gradually increase the duration as you become more comfortable with the practice. Remember, the goal is to remain present and aware, not to achieve any particular outcome or distance.

Another critical aspect of global mindfulness practices is the role of collaboration in fostering exploration and community support for healing. Collaborative practices, such as group meditation sessions, yoga classes, or mindfulness workshops, create spaces where individuals can explore different techniques in a supportive environment. These gatherings are opportunities for sharing experiences, learning new methods, and building connections with others facing similar challenges. The collective energy and shared intentions of the group can amplify the benefits of mindfulness, enhancing motivation and commitment to personal growth and healing.

Through collaborative practices, individuals are encouraged to engage with various mindfulness exercises, ranging from silent meditation to expressive arts therapies, facilitating a broader understanding of mindfulness. Such exploration allows people to find practices that resonate with their unique experiences and needs, leading to more personalized and effective pain management strategies. Moreover, the communal aspect of these practices strengthens social bonds, reducing feelings of isolation and fostering a network of emotional support.

Cultural Sensitivity in Healing

In today's interconnected world, cultural sensitivity in health and pain management is essential. It acts as a bridge to more effective therapy communication and understanding, ensuring that healing practices are both inclusive and effective for patients from diverse backgrounds. When healthcare providers embrace cultural diversity, they create environments conducive to better patient interactions, fostering an atmosphere where healing is perceived as a mutual journey rather than a one-sided process.

One critical aspect of culturally sensitive care is the ability to communicate effectively across cultural boundaries. Understanding that patients come with their own set of cultural beliefs and values can significantly enhance therapeutic relationships. For instance, according to Anandarajah et al.,

(2016), integrating spiritual care training into medical curricula helped practitioners understand how culture influences patient perceptions, thereby improving provider-patient communication (Givler & Maani-Fogelman, 2023). By acknowledging cultural differences, healthcare providers can tailor communication strategies, bridging potential gaps caused by misunderstandings and creating a foundation for trust and openness.

Furthermore, tailoring approaches that respect cultural contexts significantly improve patient engagement. Customized care plans that honor a patient's cultural background not only increase participation in treatment but also bolster adherence to medical advice. This personalization is key, as it acknowledges the patient's identity and health beliefs. In cases where language barriers exist, ensuring access to interpreters or bilingual staff becomes paramount. According to Yelton and Jildeh (2023), utilizing professional interpreters mitigates miscommunications that often arise when relying on family members or nonverbal cues. Such efforts affirm to patients that their cultural identity is valued, encouraging them to engage more fully in their treatment plans.

The role of healthcare providers extends beyond personal interaction; it involves building a culturally competent system within healthcare settings. Providers trained in cultural competence are better equipped to recognize and address disparities that patients face due to systemic biases. These professionals strive to dismantle these barriers, enabling equitable treatment outcomes. As highlighted by Dogan et al. (Yelton & Jildeh, 2023), many physiotherapists report significant challenges when treating culturally diverse populations. However, continuous education and training in cultural competence can empower therapists and physicians to provide equal and just care, thus strengthening the rapport between healthcare systems and minority communities.

Ethical considerations play a crucial role in fostering mutual respect and guiding informed healing journeys. Respecting a patient's cultural norms means involving them in decision-making processes concerning their treatment, which is an integral part of ethical medical practice. Patients who feel heard and respected are likelier to trust healthcare recommendations, enhancing cooperation throughout their care journey. Moreover, ethical practice ensures that choices align with patients' cultural values, minimizing potential conflicts between medical interventions and personal beliefs.

Guidelines for tailoring approaches that reinforce cultural sensitivity in healthcare are vital. Firstly, healthcare teams should assess the cultural dimensions of the communities they serve. This involves acknowledging different health beliefs, practices, languages, and traditions. Secondly, incorporating cultural competence into continuing medical education programs can elevate practitioners' understanding of diverse health narratives. Finally, institutional policies should promote inclusivity and representation in healthcare leadership roles, ensuring that decision-making includes diverse perspectives.

Implementing these guidelines not only addresses immediate health concerns but also plants the seed for long-term improvements in patient satisfaction and health outcomes. Consider the findings presented by Cruz-Oliver et al. (2017) in their evaluation of culturally sensitive end-of-life care – recognizing cultural nuances allowed healthcare providers to administer more compassionate and appropriate care, facilitating better experiences for patients and their families (Givler & Maani-Fogelman, 2023).

Through collaborative efforts, healthcare professionals can transform the landscape of pain management into one characterized by empathy and understanding. Patients benefit from the assurance that their cultural identity is respected and integrated into their care. Furthermore, this approach fosters a holistic perspective on healing, one that transcends mere physical well-being and encompasses emotional and cultural dimensions of health.

Lessons from Indigenous Cultures

Indigenous pain and healing practices offer a wealth of insights for those seeking alternative methods to manage chronic pain. By exploring these traditional approaches, we uncover a tapestry of wisdom that emphasizes the integration of mind, body, and spirit, fostering a holistic perspective on wellness.

Holistic Healing Approaches

One of the profound lessons from indigenous cultures is their commitment to holistic health, which honors the interconnectedness of mind, body, and spirit. Unlike Western medicine, which often focuses primarily on symptomatic relief, indigenous practices consider the totality of an individual's experience. This means recognizing the natural cycles of life and understanding how they impact well-being. For instance, many Native American traditions view pain not just as a physical ailment but also as a disruption in personal harmony and balance with nature (Koithan & Farrell, 2010). Such perspectives encourage an exploration of non-physical factors contributing to pain, inviting individuals to look beyond immediate relief and seek deeper alignment with the self and the environment.

As chronic conditions often lie at the intersection of physical, emotional, and spiritual distress, incorporating these ideas can lead to more comprehensive healing strategies. Indigenous teachings remind us that the healing process is dynamic, requiring attention to inner rhythms and environmental influences, thus promoting a more sustainable approach to health.

Rituals and Traditions

Community involvement and spirituality are central to indigenous healing rituals. These ceremonies engage not only the individual but also family members and the wider community. For example, Native American healing ceremonies may last days or weeks, filled with songs, prayers, and dances, creating a collective energy believed to enhance the healing process (Cohen, 2006). This emphasis on shared experiences builds a sense of belonging, which is often missing in modern medical settings where treatments can feel isolating.

For readers seeking alternative pain management techniques, incorporating communal rituals could be transformative. Whether it's through participation in group meditation, prayer circles, or supportive gatherings, these activities provide both emotional support and a reaffirmation of one's place within a community. Such practices serve not only to alleviate pain but also to strengthen spiritual connections, enhancing overall well-being. In this context, it is important to acknowledge cultural differences and adapt practices respectfully, ensuring genuine engagement rather than superficial adoption.

Elders and Wisdom Keepers

In indigenous societies, elders hold a revered status, serving as keepers of ancestral knowledge. Their insights are invaluable in understanding traditional healing methods. Unlike the often youth-oriented focus of Western culture, indigenous communities prioritize the wisdom of elders, drawing on their experiences to guide younger generations in maintaining health and balance (Lee, 2024). This highlights the importance of respecting and learning from those who have navigated similar challenges before us.

Engaging with elders can provide a richer understanding of pain and its roots, offering guidance that extends beyond clinical diagnoses. Their stories and teachings offer perspectives that emphasize patience, perseverance, and a deep understanding of the human condition. For those exploring alternative pain management, seeking out such wisdom can foster personal growth and a greater appreciation for the healing journey as a lifelong path.

Nature and Healing

Finally, indigenous practices underscore the essential role of nature in healing. Traditional beliefs affirm that the natural world holds powerful restorative properties, reinforcing the connection between the mind and body. Engaging with nature—whether through herbal remedies, immersion in natural landscapes, or simply observing seasonal changes—can enhance the healing process. Native American practices often involve ceremonies that align with the seasons, celebrating harvests or making offerings at dawn, thereby attuning participants to the earth's rhythms (Koithan & Farrell, 2010).

Incorporating elements of nature into one's daily routine can serve as a potent reminder of our place within the broader ecosystem. Simple acts like walking in green spaces, meditating outdoors, or using plant-based therapies can rejuvenate the spirit and alleviate stress-related pain, promoting a harmonious balance between internal states and the external environment.

Guidelines for Incorporating Nature into Healing

To integrate nature effectively into your healing routine, consider these practices:

Daily Nature Walks: Spend time walking in natural settings and pay attention to the sights, sounds, and scents around you. This presence can reduce stress and encourage mindfulness.

Herbal Remedies: Explore the use of herbs known for their therapeutic properties, following guidance from knowledgeable practitioners to ensure safe usage.

Seasonal Observances: Acknowledge seasonal changes through simple rituals or reflections that realign you with the earth's cycles, fostering a sense of unity with the natural world.

Final Insights

In examining the diverse cultural perspectives on pain and healing, this chapter has revealed a rich tapestry of approaches that extend beyond the physical into the realms of mind and spirit. From Eastern philosophies that emphasize the flow of vital energy like Qi, to Ayurvedic traditions seeking balance through personalized practices, these views offer holistic ways to address pain. We've delved into how mindfulness, with its roots in both Eastern and Western traditions, empowers individuals to manage their pain by fostering awareness and acceptance. This introspection not only alters one's relationship with pain but also nurtures emotional resilience and mental clarity. Community rituals and shared experiences further accentuate the power of connectivity in healing, reminding us that we are never alone in our journey toward wellness.

As we embrace these insights, it becomes clear that integrating cultural wisdom into modern pain management can transform the experience for those living with chronic conditions. Indigenous teachings, Western medical advancements, and cross-cultural mindfulness techniques together form an inclusive landscape where each individual's unique path is honored. By recognizing the importance of spiritual, emotional, and community factors, we nurture a more profound connection to ourselves and those around us. Ultimately, this chapter encourages readers to explore these diverse practices with an open heart, finding comfort and empowerment in approaches that honor their personal stories and needs. As we continue this journey towards healing, may compassion, understanding, and shared humanity guide us all.

Reference List

AlSubaie, Aeishaa AlSubaie, Bajawi, Zahra Awaji, Hassan, A., Shabani, K. M., Ibrahim, S. A., Nasser, A., Owaid, M., Khalaf, H., Alhamadan, Fahad Hamadan, Al-Qahtani, Atef Fahid Ayed, Aldhafeeri, Tahani Huwaydi, Aldhafeeri, Mashael Huwaydi, Abdullah, A. I., Mubarak, A.-S. N., & Mohammed.

(2024, December). *Integrating Mindfulness-Based Interventions into Mental Health Nursing: A Review of Evidence, Biochemical Mechanisms, and Implementation Challenges.* Journal of Medicinal and Chemical Sciences; Sami Publishing Company (SPC). https://doi.org/10.26655/JMCHEMSCI.2024.12.8

Elendu, C. (2024, July 12). *The evolution of ancient healing practices: From shamanism to Hippocratic medicine: A review.* Medicine. https://doi.org/10.1097/MD.0000000000039005

Givler, A., & Maani-Fogelman, P. A. (2023). *The importance of cultural competence in pain and palliative care.* National Library of Medicine; StatPearls Publishing. https://www.ncbi.nlm.nih.gov/books/NBK493154/

Hofmann, S. G., & Gómez, A. F. (2018). *Mindfulness-Based Interventions for Anxiety and Depression.* Psychiatric Clinics of North America. https://doi.org/10.1016/j.psc.2017.08.008

Ikigai Transfromations- Live on Purpose. (2024). Apple Podcasts. https://podcasts.apple.com/pe/podcast/ikigai-transfromations-live-on-purpose/id1591691354

Kriakous, S. A., Elliott, K. A., Lamers, C., & Owen, R. (2021, September 24). *The effectiveness of mindfulness-based stress reduction on the psychological functioning of healthcare professionals: A systematic review.* Mindfulness. https://doi.org/10.1007/s12671-020-01500-9

Koithan, M., & Farrell, C. (2010, June 1). *Indigenous Native American Healing Traditions.* The Journal for Nurse Practitioners; National Library of Medicine. https://doi.org/10.1016/j.nurpra.2010.03.016

Lee, C. (2024, April 24). *Healing Ourselves as Indigenous People*. Www.aft.org. https://www.aft.org/hc/spring2024/lee

Schuman-Olivier, Z., Trombka, M., Lovas, D. A., Brewer, J. A., Vago, D. R., Gawande, R., Dunne, J. P., Lazar, S. W., Loucks, E. B., & Fulwiler, C. (2020). *Mindfulness and behavior change*. Harvard Review of Psychiatry. https://doi.org/10.1097/HRP.0000000000000277

Yelton, M. J., & Jildeh, T. R. (2023, May 23). *Cultural Competence and the Postoperative Experience: Pain Control and Rehabilitation*. Arthroscopy, Sports Medicine, and Rehabilitation. https://doi.org/10.1016/j.asmr.2023.04.016

CHAPTER 15

Long-term Benefits of Mindfulness Practice

Practicing mindfulness can be a transformative journey toward improving one's life, especially when dealing with persistent pain. Mindfulness is an approach that encourages individuals to pay close attention to their emotions and experiences, fostering a sense of calmness and presence. By focusing on the now, mindfulness allows practitioners to move beyond discomfort and discover new perspectives on managing challenges. As you embark on this exploration, you'll begin to uncover how sustained mindfulness can shape your perception of pain and enhance daily living.

This chapter delves into the long-term benefits of adopting mindfulness as part of your routine. It will explore various aspects such as emotional balance, reduced reliance on medication, and improved interpersonal relationships. You'll discover how regular mindfulness practice contributes to mental resilience and better equips individuals to handle stressors. Through evidence-based discussions and practical insights, the chapter offers valuable strategies for embracing mindfulness as a tool for achieving a more harmonious lifestyle amid chronic pain. As you read on, you'll find a comprehensive understanding of how mindfulness can be integrated into daily life, providing not only relief but also a path to a more fulfilling existence.

Sustained Well-being

Long-term mindfulness practice has a profound impact on one's overall well-being and quality of life, particularly for individuals dealing with chronic pain. By nurturing mental balance, mindfulness opens pathways towards resilience, tranquility, and deeper interpersonal relationships, all of which contribute to healthier living.

Engaging in regular mindfulness practice can significantly reduce symptoms of depression and anxiety. According to Keng et al. (2011), mindfulness encourages an acceptance-based approach to thoughts and emotions, allowing individuals to develop a more adaptive relationship with negative experiences. Over time, this practice diminishes the intensity and frequency of depressive and anxious episodes by promoting emotional awareness and reducing rumination. The work of Lykins and Baer (2009) emphasizes how experienced meditators often report lower levels of psychological distress compared to non-meditators, underscoring the value of consistent mindfulness engagement.

Physiological benefits are equally noteworthy. Studies have shown that regular mindfulness practices can help lower blood pressure and heart rate, contributing to cardiovascular health. This is crucial for those managing chronic pain, as stress-induced hypertension can exacerbate physical symptoms. Mindfulness practices such as focused breathing and meditation promote relaxation responses that counteract stress-induced physiological arousal, resulting in more stable blood pressure and improved heart health (Mental Health Foundation, 2022).

Furthermore, mindfulness appears to be linked to healthier aging through its positive effects on immune function. Chronic stress weakens the immune system, leaving individuals more susceptible to illnesses. Mindfulness, however, fosters recovery and resilience by enhancing the body's response to stress. Techniques like body scanning and mindful breathing increase parasympathetic nervous system activity, which supports immunity. The findings suggest that those engaging in mindfulness experience fewer age-related declines in immune function, potentially extending their healthy years (Keng et al., 2011).

Interpersonal relationships also benefit from long-term mindfulness engagement. Enhanced empathy and communication skills emerge as individuals become more attuned to their own emotions and those of others. Mindfulness promotes active listening and presence, essential components for meaningful connections. As empathy deepens, so does the ability to navigate conflicts with patience and understanding. These improvements in social interactions lead to more robust support networks, which are vital for coping with chronic pain challenges (Mental Health Foundation, 2022).

Regular mindfulness practice encourages healthier coping mechanisms for stress. By integrating mindfulness into daily routines, individuals learn to respond to stressful situations calmly rather than reactively. This practice shifts focus from immediate stressors to a broader perspective, enabling individuals to manage their stress more effectively and maintain a sense of equilibrium despite life's ups and downs. With continued practice, mindfulness equips individuals with tools to face adversity with a poised and centered mindset, fostering inner strength and adaptability.

Moreover, mindfulness cultivates a more positive outlook on life despite chronic pain challenges. A mindful approach encourages gratitude and appreciation for the present moment, shifting attention away from discomfort or dissatisfaction. By embracing mindfulness, individuals cultivate an accepting attitude towards their pain and limitations, thus reducing suffering associated with resistance. This shift in perception allows for more moments of joy and contentment, ultimately enhancing quality of life.

For individuals seeking to integrate mindfulness into their lives, it begins with setting aside even a few minutes each day for meditation or mindful breathing. Guided sessions, whether through in-person classes, apps, or online resources, provide a structured path towards building a consistent practice. It's important to remember that mindfulness is a personal journey; there's no right way to do it, and everyone can find their unique rhythm.

Chronic Pain Management Improvements

Sustained mindfulness practice can have a profound impact on long-term pain management strategies, offering an alternate path to handling chronic pain. By leveraging the power of attention and awareness, mindfulness practitioners experience a shift in focus from pain sensations, which can significantly reduce perceived pain levels (Zeidan & Vago, 2016).

By using techniques such as mindfulness of breath and open-monitoring meditation, individuals learn to observe their pain without becoming overwhelmed by it. This practice involves acknowledging the sensation of pain without attaching a negative emotional response or judgment to it. For example, consider someone experiencing chronic back pain. Instead of fixating on the discomfort, they might direct their awareness towards their breathing, allowing the immediate pain sensations to exist without dominating their conscious experience.

Mindfulness also provides tools for effectively managing pain flare-ups. Techniques such as body scan meditation and loving-kindness meditation equip individuals with methods to cope with intense episodes of pain. When a flare-up occurs, rather than succumbing to panic or distress, a person trained in mindfulness can employ these practices to stay grounded. This approach not only helps in reducing immediate suffering but teaches how to handle future instances with greater composure.

Moreover, integrating mindfulness with self-care practices creates a holistic approach that reduces dependency on medication. Many chronic pain sufferers rely heavily on pharmaceuticals to manage their conditions, often facing undesirable side effects. Combining mindfulness with lifestyle adjustments, such as regular physical activity, balanced nutrition, and adequate rest, can create a comprehensive strategy that diminishes reliance on medication. The 8-week mindfulness-based stress reduction (MBSR) program has shown promising results in this regard, where participants reported improved quality of life and decreased medication use after adopting mindfulness practices (Hilton et al., 2017).

Resilience against pain-related stressors is another significant benefit developed through regular mindfulness practice. Mindfulness nurtures mental fortitude by fostering an attitude of acceptance and patience. As individuals consistently engage in mindful practices, they build a kind of psychological armor, enhancing their ability to withstand the adversities that come with chronic pain. This resilience doesn't eliminate pain but transforms one's relationship with it, making it more manageable and less intrusive in daily life.

The journey towards incorporating mindfulness into one's life requires dedication and patience, yet the rewards are substantial. By gradually shifting focus away from the debilitating aspects of pain, individuals gain control over their experiences. They move from being at the mercy of their condition to living alongside it with increased agency and peace.

To illustrate the effectiveness of mindfulness in pain management, consider evidence from various clinical studies. For instance, research has shown that chronic pain patients who practice mindfulness report significant reductions in pain intensity and improvements in emotional well-being. These findings suggest that the mental clarity and emotional equilibrium fostered through mindfulness play pivotal roles in reshaping one's perception of pain.

In addition to personal anecdotes, scientific research supports these claims. Neuroimaging studies reveal changes in brain structures related to pain perception following consistent mindfulness practice. The posterior cingulate cortex, involved in self-referential processing, is one of the areas affected. These changes indicate a rewiring of neural pathways, leading to a more adaptable experience of pain.

While the integration of mindfulness into traditional healthcare settings is still developing, its potential is being increasingly recognized. As more individuals turn to this ancient practice, mindfulness is finding its place among modern therapeutic approaches. Although further research is needed to establish standardized protocols, the existing evidence underscores mindfulness as a viable adjunctive therapy for chronic pain management.

For those beginning their journey on this path, it is important to approach mindfulness with realistic expectations. The benefits are cumulative and may take time to manifest fully. Regular engagement is key, as is the willingness to persist even when progress seems slow. By maintaining consistency, individuals can unlock the transformative impacts of mindfulness on their pain experiences.

Longevity and Mindfulness

Mindfulness, often regarded as a holistic approach to well-being, also plays a vital role in enhancing lifespan. At its most fundamental level, mindfulness encourages one to remain present, fostering an awareness that can subtly influence physical health and longevity. The intricate interplay between mindfulness and lifespan begins with the cellular components of our bodies, specifically telomeres. Telomeres are protective caps at the ends of chromosomes and serve as markers of biological aging. Research has shown that engaging in mindfulness practices may contribute to the preservation of telomere length.

Telomeres naturally shorten over time due to cell division. However, factors such as chronic stress can accelerate this process, leading to premature cellular aging. Mindfulness, with its potential for stress reduction, offers a buffer against this acceleration. Studies, including those conducted by researchers like Blackburn (2005), suggest that individuals practicing mindfulness exhibit longer telomeres, indicative of slower cellular aging. By mitigating stress's impact, mindfulness may support better maintenance of these protective chromosomal endcaps, promoting healthier aging.

Beyond cellular benefits, mindfulness practice is linked to reduced inflammation. Chronic inflammation is a common pathway to several diseases, such as cardiovascular ailments and autoimmune disorders. Mindful practices, including meditation and focused breathing, may help modulate inflammatory responses. This modulation is crucial because excessive inflammation contributes to various life-shortening conditions. Research backed by findings from studies like West et al. (2022) indicates that mindfulness interventions can alter gene expression related to inflammation, thereby offering protective effects against the cascade of harmful health outcomes associated with it.

Social connections are another pivotal element that ties mindfulness to extended lifespan. Humans are inherently social creatures, and the quality of our interactions significantly impacts our health. Mindfulness practices foster greater empathy and communication skills, which enhance interpersonal relationships. These improved social interactions provide robust support networks that can act as stress buffers, promoting longevity. For instance, research shows that individuals with strong social ties have longer telomeres and lower levels of stress hormones. Creating intentional spaces for mindful communication strengthens relationships, leading to increased life satisfaction and potentially longer lives.

Moreover, cross-cultural mindfulness programs serve as a powerful tool for promoting health equity, particularly in underserved communities. Such programs emphasize inclusivity and accessibility, ensuring that individuals from diverse backgrounds can benefit from mindfulness practices. These programs often focus on adapting traditional mindfulness techniques to fit cultural contexts, making them more relatable and impactful. In doing so, they address disparities in health resources and education, offering hope for improved community health outcomes. The inclusive nature of these initiatives can lead to widespread adoption, ultimately contributing to enhanced longevity across varied demographic groups.

Encouraging lifestyle changes through mindfulness remains essential for both physical and emotional health. By promoting balance, mindfulness helps individuals cultivate habits that support overall well-being. Incorporating mindfulness into daily routines—whether through meditation, mindful eating, or exercise—encourages healthier choices that cumulatively extend lifespan. As mindfulness becomes an integral aspect of one's lifestyle, it fosters resilience, equipping individuals with tools to navigate life's challenges with grace and patience.

In summary, while practicing mindfulness, one embarks on a journey that intricately weaves together various aspects of life, all contributing to prolonged longevity. From supporting cellular vitality through telomere preservation to reducing systemic inflammation, mindfulness exerts a profound influence on physical health. Strengthened social bonds and culturally responsive mindfulness programs further underscore its comprehensive benefits. These practices build bridges across communities, narrowing health disparities and fostering a more balanced, harmonious existence.

Mindfulness and Aging

Mindfulness is an invaluable tool for promoting healthier aging. As individuals age, several physical and cognitive challenges arise that can significantly impact their quality of life. However, the practice of mindfulness offers various benefits that contribute positively to the process of aging. One of the prominent advantages is the enhancement of memory and attention span among seniors. Regular engagement in mindfulness practices encourages individuals to focus on the present moment, which in turn helps sharpen cognitive functions like memory recall and attention to detail. According to research, seniors who incorporate mindfulness into their daily routines often experience notable improvements in these areas, thereby maintaining mental acuity as they age (Dr. Kirilyuk Inna Anatolyivna, 2023).

The acceptance of aging-related challenges is another key aspect where mindfulness plays a crucial role. Emotional resilience is a vital part of navigating the complexities of growing older. By embracing mindfulness, seniors learn to accept the natural progression of life without dwelling on past regrets or becoming anxious about the future. This acceptance fosters emotional resilience, enabling older adults to cope with the physical and emotional changes that come with age. Mindfulness teaches individuals to observe their thoughts and emotions without judgment, allowing for greater emotional balance and reduced stress levels. This skill becomes particularly important when confronting age-related issues such as retirement, loss of loved ones, or changing health conditions.

In addition to mental and emotional benefits, mindfulness also impacts physical health, specifically in maintaining joint health through mindful movement practices. For many seniors, maintaining mobility is essential for independence and overall well-being. Encouraging activities like yoga or tai chi, which integrate mindfulness into movement, can help preserve joint flexibility and strength. These practices emphasize gentle, deliberate movements that promote awareness of the body, helping to prevent injuries and alleviate chronic pain often associated with arthritis and other age-related conditions. Such mindful movement encourages seniors to stay active while minimizing strain on the body (<i>The Power of a Holistic Approach to Aging</i>, 2024).

Community engagement is another area where mindfulness contributes to healthier aging. Isolation is a significant concern for older adults, often leading to feelings of loneliness and depression. By participating in mindfulness-based community gatherings or classes, seniors have the opportunity to connect with others who share similar interests and challenges. This sense of belonging not only combats isolation but also provides a support system that enhances emotional and mental well-being. Engaging with peers in mindfulness activities allows older adults to share experiences, learn from one another, and build meaningful relationships, ultimately reducing the risk of social isolation and its associated health effects.

To maximize the benefits of mindfulness for healthier aging, consistency in practice is crucial. Developing a routine where mindfulness integrates seamlessly into daily life can create a sense of stability and control over one's well-being. For example, setting aside specific times each day for meditation or engaging in mindful movement exercises can establish mindfulness as a foundational habit affecting overall lifestyle choices. By embedding mindfulness into their routine, seniors are likely to experience sustained improvements in mental clarity, emotional regulation, and physical health over time.

Furthermore, encouraging seniors to explore different mindfulness techniques is important. Since mindfulness is a versatile practice, individuals may find certain methods more appealing or effective than others. Offering exposure to various mindfulness strategies, such as breathing exercises, visualization, or guided meditations, can help seniors identify what resonates with them personally. This personalized approach ensures that mindfulness remains engaging and beneficial for each individual's unique preferences and needs.

Future Implications of Mindfulness Research

Mindfulness, long practiced in contemplative traditions, is increasingly recognized for its potential within healthcare settings to support a holistic approach to pain management and overall health. As medical communities explore integrative practices, the integration of mindfulness into healthcare can be a pivotal shift. By treating patients not just physically but also emotionally and mentally, healthcare professionals enable a more comprehensive path to wellness. Mindfulness techniques can work alongside traditional treatments to foster self-awareness and emotional resilience, teaching patients how to navigate chronic pain without being overwhelmed by it (Fritz et al., 2022).

Current research highlights that mindfulness has distinct benefits by shifting focus from emotional reactions to sensory perceptions, reducing the intensity and unpleasantness of chronic pain (Zeidan et al., 2019). Future research is poised to tailor mindfulness interventions towards specific populations, acknowledging differences across age, gender, or health conditions. Designing studies that address these nuances will enhance the efficacy of mindfulness practices, offering personalized care plans that meet unique needs and improve patient outcomes.

On a global scale, mindfulness movements are adapting these practices for cultural relevance, ensuring they resonate with diverse groups. This adaptability is crucial in making mindfulness accessible and relatable worldwide. For instance, incorporating culturally significant elements into mindfulness practice can deepen engagement and acceptance, breaking down barriers to participation across various communities. These adaptations not only honor cultural diversity but also enrich the practice by integrating different perspectives and traditions.

Moreover, committing to lifelong mindfulness practices fosters holistic thinking that extends beyond immediate health benefits. This commitment nurtures an individual's ability to approach health from a multidimensional perspective, considering emotional, psychological, and social well-being. Over time, this holistic thinking encourages a broader view of health that integrates lifestyle choices, stress management, and interpersonal relationships, ultimately supporting a balanced life. Engaging fully with mindfulness provides individuals with tools to enhance their quality of life by promoting inner peace and resilience.

To cultivate enhanced coping mechanisms, individuals are encouraged to integrate daily mindfulness exercises such as body scan meditation or mindful breathing into their routines. These practices help develop awareness and acceptance of present experiences, providing effective strategies to deal with pain flare-ups and stress-related situations. Such techniques empower individuals to respond thoughtfully rather than react impulsively, fostering a sense of control over challenging situations.

Additionally, as mindfulness practices become more entrenched, there is potential for less reliance on medication. This does not diminish the role of pharmaceuticals but rather complements them, offering alternative means to manage pain and reduce dependency on medications. Practitioners can apply mindfulness to alleviate symptoms, mitigate emotional distress associated with pain, and diminish habitual responses like excessive medication use (Fritz et al., 2022). In doing so, patients might experience fewer side effects and improved overall well-being.

Long-term mindfulness practitioners often report profound adaptations that extend into many facets of life. Through consistent practice, mindfulness promotes cognitive restructuring, encouraging individuals to perceive their circumstances with greater clarity and equanimity. It's vital to note that developing mindfulness takes patience and persistence, but the rewards, such as enduring peace and resilience against life's demands, make it a worthy investment. These adaptations can lead to improved decision-making, better emotional regulation, and enhanced interpersonal relationships.

Insights and Implications

In this chapter, we've journeyed through the remarkable ways mindfulness can transform the lives of those experiencing chronic pain. Mindfulness opens a new world of possibilities by fostering an environment of awareness and acceptance. It allows individuals to reframe their relationship with pain, diminishing its hold on their daily experiences. With consistent practice, techniques like focused breathing and body scanning become powerful tools in reducing stress and anxiety. These practices not only facilitate emotional resilience but also empower individuals to face each day with renewed strength and calm.

As we've explored, integrating mindfulness into one's life is more than just managing physical symptoms—it's about nurturing a holistic sense of well-being. By embracing mindfulness, individuals unlock the potential for healthier lifestyle choices, improved interpersonal relationships, and even a brighter outlook on life. While the journey requires patience and perseverance, it offers profound rewards: a life enriched by moments of peace, gratitude, and connection. For anyone seeking solace amid chronic pain, mindfulness provides a gentle path forward, promising both healing and hope.

Reference List

Dr. Kirilyuk Inna Anatolyivna. (2023, April 3). *The Many Benefits Of Meditation and Mindfulness For Seniors.* Megawecare; Mega We Care. https://www.megawecare.com/good-health-by-yourself/healthy-aging/meditation-for-seniors

Fritz, J. M., Rhon, D. I., Garland, E. L., Hanley, A. W., Greenlee, T. A., Fino, N. F., Martin, B. I., Highland, K. B., & Greene, T. (2022, September 7). *The Effectiveness of a Mindfulness-Based Intervention Integrated with Physical Therapy (MIND-PT) for Post-Surgical Rehabilitation after Lumbar Surgery: A Protocol for a Randomized Controlled Trial as Part of the Back Pain Consortium (BACPAC) Research Program.* https://doi.org/10.1093/pm/pnac138

Hilton, L., Hempel, S., Ewing, B. A., Apaydin, E., Xenakis, L., Newberry, S., Colaiaco, B., Maher, A. R., Shanman, R. M., Sorbero, M. E., & Maglione, M. A. (2017, September 22). *Mindfulness meditation for chronic pain: Systematic review and meta-analysis*. Annals of Behavioral Medicine. https://doi.org/10.1007/s12160-016-9844-2

Keng, S. L., Smoski, M. J., & Robins, C. J. (2011). *Effects of Mindfulness on Psychological health: a Review of Empirical Studies*. Clinical Psychology Review. https://doi.org/10.1016/j.cpr.2011.04.006

Mental Health Foundation. (2022). *How to look after your mental health using mindfulness*. Www.mentalhealth.org.uk. https://www.mentalhealth.org.uk/explore-mental-health/publications/how-look-after-your-mental-health-using-mindfulness

Puterman, E., & Epel, E. (2012, November). *An Intricate Dance: Life Experience, Multisystem Resiliency, and Rate of Telomere Decline Throughout the Lifespan*. Social and Personality Psychology Compass. https://doi.org/10.1111/j.1751-9004.2012.00465.x

The Power of a Holistic Approach to Aging. (2024). Humancareny.com. https://www.humancareny.com/blog/holistic-approach-to-aging

West, T. N., Zhou, J., Brantley, M. M., Kim, S. L., Brantley, J., Salzberg, S., Cole, S. W., & Fredrickson, B. L. (2022, March 16). *Effect of Mindfulness Versus Loving-kindness Training on Leukocyte Gene Expression in Midlife Adults Raised in Low-Socioeconomic Status Households*. Mindfulness. https://doi.org/10.1007/s12671-022-01857-z

Zeidan, F., & Vago, D. R. (2016, June). *Mindfulness meditation-based pain relief: a mechanistic account*. Annals of the New York Academy of Sciences. https://doi.org/10.1111/nyas.13153

Zeidan, F., Baumgartner, J. N., & Coghill, R. C. (2019). *The neural mechanisms of mindfulness-based pain relief.* PAIN Reports. https://doi.org/10.1097/pr9.0000000000000759

CHAPTER 16

Embracing a Mindful Life

Embracing a mindful life involves taking small, intentional steps toward integrating mindfulness into every aspect of our existence. This journey, especially for those managing chronic pain, is about more than just finding relief; it's about unlocking deeper fulfillment and aligning daily actions with what truly matters. Living mindfully means looking at each moment not just as it happens but as an opportunity to connect with our values and inner peace. Mindfulness invites us to see beyond the immediate discomfort and recognize the potential for growth and transformation that lies in every challenge. As you embark on this exploration, consider how the gentle yet profound practice of mindfulness can illuminate paths towards a more fulfilling and purpose-driven life.

In this chapter, you'll discover the transformative power of incorporating mindfulness into various facets of your life, helping you build resilience and find harmony even amidst challenges. By exploring value-driven living, you'll gain insights into identifying what truly matters to you, allowing this understanding to guide your choices and actions. Through practical exercises and reflections, you'll learn how setting intentions can shape your day positively, fostering motivation and alignment with your core beliefs. Additionally, the chapter delves into acceptance, empowering you to embrace pain without letting it overshadow your life's purpose. Within these pages lies a roadmap to intentionally weaving mindfulness throughout your daily routine, creating lasting change and enhancing your overall quality of life.

Mindfulness and Purpose

Embracing a mindful life, especially when living with chronic pain, involves recognizing how mindfulness can enhance fulfillment and align our daily actions with personal values. The challenge of chronic pain often clouds judgment, making everyday decisions overwhelming. However, identifying personal values becomes a beacon, guiding us through this murkiness. When we understand what truly matters, we gain clarity that simplifies decision-making, allowing us to choose paths that resonate with our deepest beliefs. Identifying these values is integral to achieving a purposeful life despite the ongoing struggle with pain.

When deciding which values to prioritize, it's helpful to reflect on moments in our lives where we felt most alive or deeply satisfied. This reflection sheds light on the principles that are crucial to who we are. By organizing these moments, we develop a tapestry of value-driven living. For instance, if kindness and community are cherished values, then engaging in volunteer work might become a priority, even on days when physical discomfort is pronounced.

Aligning daily actions with these identified values fosters empowerment and motivation. It transforms passive existence into active engagement. When your actions reflect your values, you experience an inner harmony that counteracts the disruptive nature of chronic pain. For example, someone valuing creativity might set aside a few minutes each day for writing or drawing, activities that not only distract from pain but also reaffirm their identity and passions. Thus, every small action aligned with values contributes to creating a richer, more meaningful life.

Mindfulness plays a pivotal role in shifting our perspective towards challenges, viewing them as opportunities for growth rather than insurmountable obstacles. Chronic pain is often seen as an antagonist, but mindfulness teaches us to reframe it as a teacher. Through acceptance, we learn resilience, nurturing a mindset that welcomes growth. Mindfulness encourages us to pause and observe our reactions without judgment during painful episodes. Rather than resisting pain, acknowledging it allows us to explore new coping mechanisms and insights into our emotional responses.

This approach is supported by Acceptance and Commitment Therapy (ACT), which promotes psychological flexibility—the ability to adapt to changing circumstances while maintaining alignment with our values (CIFI, 2024). ACT's emphasis on mindfulness equips individuals with tools to navigate life's stressors without becoming immobilized by them. Viewing pain through this lens fosters resilience, enabling us to see beyond immediate discomfort to a future filled with possibilities.

Living intentionally is fundamental to increasing presence and aligning with one's purpose. Establishing routines that reflect chosen values supports consistency and reduces anxiety about daily choices. Intentional living revolves around embedding mindfulness in our routines, allowing each moment, whether mundane or significant, to be anchored in awareness. Setting clear intentions at the beginning of each day—such as choosing gratitude over frustration or opting for patience instead of hasty reactions—creates a roadmap for fulfilling days.

One practical way to integrate intentional living is through routine-building exercises. A morning ritual that includes meditation or simple affirmations can center the mind before engaging with the day's challenges. These practices need not be lengthy; even brief moments of mindfulness can set a positive tone. This practice enhances presence throughout the day, helping us engage fully with tasks at hand and fostering a deeper connection to our purpose.

Guidelines for enhancing purpose through mindful living include establishing a daily routine that aligns with personal values, practicing mindfulness exercises, and regularly reflecting on progress. By committing to this holistic approach, the journey of living with chronic pain becomes less daunting and more empowering.

ACT provides practical strategies for cultivating such skills, aiding individuals in gaining a deeper understanding of their chronic pain. Its techniques emphasize the importance of living aligned with values, reducing distress and increasing overall quality of life (*Acceptance and Commitment Therapy Los Angeles | ACT Psychology*, 2020). Utilizing these methods, we gain the ability to manage not only physical symptoms but also emotional well-being.

Creating a Vision for Healing

Imagining a future free of chronic pain may seem distant, but envisioning healing is a potent first step towards transformation. By visualizing specific goals, your path to well-being becomes clearer and more attainable. This process begins with a tool known as a vision board—an artistic collection that truly embodies your aspirations.

Vision boards serve as a visual reminder of the goals we set for ourselves, providing a daily dose of inspiration. For individuals living with chronic pain, creating a vision board can help clarify healing goals, anchoring them in tangible images and words. It's about taking those abstract desires—such as finding relief or regaining mobility—and representing them visually. This method has proven powerful in various scenarios (AFFiNE, 2025). Imagine filling your board with pictures of activities you once loved but have found challenging, quotes that inspire hope, or even images depicting peace and comfort. As Madison's story illustrates, the act of visualization shouldn't be underestimated (<i>What to Put on a Vision Board: Unlock Your Goals with These 10 Inspiring Ideas | AFFiNE</i>, 2025).

Once this visual foundation is laid, it's time to refine objectives using SMART goal-setting strategies—a framework that turns dreams into actionable tasks. SMART stands for Specific, Measurable, Achievable, Relevant, and Time-bound, and it guides the creation of clear, attainable goals. Begin by specifying what you want to achieve in your healing journey, like reducing flare-ups or increasing physical activity levels. Then measure progress through journal entries documenting symptoms or milestones reached. Ensure your goals are realistic within your current capacity, allowing room for gradual improvement. Relevance keeps your goals aligned with your broader purpose: improving life quality despite chronic pain. Lastly, attach timelines to these goals. Short-term deadlines bolster motivation while longer timelines offer a pathway to larger ambitions (Brian Tracy, 2024).

Reflecting on past successes is another useful practice, providing encouragement and a resilience boost. Even if victories seem small, such as managing pain better on certain days or completing a gentle exercise routine, each success reinforces your capability to overcome challenges. Regularly reviewing these achievements can remind you of the strength you've shown, rekindling confidence when faced with setbacks.

It's about acknowledging that each step forward, no matter how tiny, is progress—a testament to what you're capable of achieving.

However, maintaining flexibility in your goals is just as crucial. Chronic pain can be unpredictable, requiring plans to adapt. Progress might not always be linear, and that's okay. Being open to modify goals in response to your body's signals prevents discouragement. Perhaps an intended daily walk is replaced with a rest day, or a new therapeutic approach is explored. The key is to remain fluid, adjusting objectives based on ongoing feedback from your body and mind. This adaptability ensures that goals remain supportive rather than overwhelming, accommodating the natural ebb and flow of your healing process while preserving a sense of agency.

Sustaining Mindfulness in Daily Life

Embracing mindfulness in every aspect of your daily life is a journey that can yield profound benefits, particularly for those managing chronic pain. By embedding mindfulness into routine activities, you cultivate resilience and create a more harmonious existence. Here are some strategies to integrate mindfulness seamlessly into your everyday experiences.

Mindful Morning Routines

Begin your day with practices that promote mindfulness, setting a positive tone for everything that follows. This foundational approach awakens your mind and body, aiding in mental clarity and overall well-being. Consider incorporating gentle stretching exercises shortly after waking up. Feel the stretch in each muscle, and breathe deeply, observing how your body responds. Similarly, when you shower, be present. Notice the warmth of the water, the scent of soap, and the sound of droplets falling. Such awareness grounds you, preparing you mentally and physically for the day ahead (How to Integrate Mindfulness into Your Everyday Life, 2023).

Another key aspect of a mindful morning is setting intentions. Spend a few minutes reflecting on what you hope to achieve. Imagine moving through your tasks calmly and efficiently. This visualization not only centers your focus but also reinforces a positive mindset. These mindful morning routines foster an environment where positivity and productivity thrive, providing a clearer path to tackle daily challenges.

Mindfulness Breaks

Throughout the day, it's beneficial to take short mindfulness breaks, especially amidst busy or stressful schedules. A few moments of intentional pause can mitigate stress and enhance your overall sense of well-being. Engage in simple practices such as deep breathing exercises. Close your eyes, inhale slowly, and exhale entirely, focusing solely on your breath's rhythm (Whitaker, 2023).

Incorporating mindful walking during breaks is another effective practice. When possible, step outside and pay attention to the sensation of your feet connecting with the ground. Notice the textures, temperatures, and sounds around you. Even brief moments spent like this can rejuvenate your mind, enabling you to return to tasks with better focus and reduced tension. These small investments in your mental health have cumulative effects, gradually enhancing your resilience against stress.

Creating Mindful Habits

Forming lasting mindful habits involves integrating them into your existing routines. This pairing ensures consistency and makes new practices easier to remember and maintain. Start by identifying a habit you already do consistently, such as drinking a cup of tea or coffee. Use these moments to become fully present. Concentrate on the taste, aroma, and warmth. Let go of other distractions and give yourself permission to enjoy the experience fully.

Similarly, establish mindful journeys on your daily commute. Instead of tuning out with music or podcasts, occasionally engage with your surroundings. Observe the landscape, notice your fellow passengers, and be aware of your thoughts and feelings as they arise. Over time, you'll find that these integrated moments of mindfulness are pervasive, naturally occurring throughout your day without need for conscious effort. They anchor you in the present, providing stability and a cultivating sense of gratitude.

Integrating Mindfulness into Routine Tasks

Everyday tasks offer abundant opportunities for practicing mindfulness, turning mundane chores into enlightening experiences. Begin by bringing mindfulness into meal preparation and consumption. Focus on each task, from selecting ingredients to savoring each bite. Pay attention to the flavors and textures, eating slowly and appreciatively. Mindful eating not only enhances your enjoyment but also encourages healthier dietary choices, potentially easing digestion-related discomforts often associated with chronic pain.

Cleaning tasks can also become mindful undertakings. Instead of rushing through chores, immerse yourself in the process. While washing dishes, feel the water temperature and the texture of each item. By engaging this way, routine tasks transform into meditative exercises that enrich your daily experience.

Technology is ever-present, but it can be utilized mindfully. Set designated times for checking emails and social media, allowing for uninterrupted focus on other tasks. During these intervals, concentrate on being present rather than distracted by screens or notifications. This mindful approach fosters better concentration, decreasing anxiety typically linked with constant connectivity.

Living Mindfully with Chronic Pain

Living with chronic pain can often feel overwhelming, but mindfulness techniques offer practical and powerful tools to manage these symptoms calmly. Mindfulness invites individuals to focus on the present moment, embracing it without judgment. This practice helps in acknowledging pain as it is, reducing its emotional weight. For instance, using mindfulness meditation, individuals are encouraged to observe their sensations rather than react with fear or frustration, allowing them to see pain more as a transient experience rather than a permanent state. This approach can significantly lessen anxiety and improve one's overall quality of life.

Incorporating mindfulness into daily routines can also help ease the burden of physical discomfort. Mindful breathing exercises can be particularly effective, providing a simple yet powerful means to manage pain. By placing attention on the breath, patients can create a tranquil mental space where they can disconnect from persistent pain signals. Additionally, practices such as guided imagery allow the mind to wander to peaceful areas, which can provide relief from the constant sensation of pain. These techniques not only alleviate immediate discomfort but also enhance emotional resilience over time, fostering a more composed response to pain flare-ups.

Acceptance plays a crucial role in managing chronic pain. The resistance to pain can be psychologically exhausting, whereas acceptance allows individuals to coexist with their discomfort without letting it rule their lives. Acknowledging pain as an unavoidable part of existence, rather than as an enemy to combat, reduces emotional distress enormously. This shift in mindset fosters resilience—an essential quality for anyone dealing with chronic conditions. Acceptance doesn't imply giving up; rather, it empowers individuals to live fully despite ongoing challenges, allowing them to focus on what truly matters in life beyond their pain (Alis, 2025).

Positive self-talk and affirmations make up another vital aspect of mindfulness practice for those experiencing chronic pain. Often, chronic pain can lead to negative self-perception, diminishing one's sense of self-worth. By consciously repeating affirmations like "I am strong" or "I trust my body," individuals can reshape their perceptions of pain. These affirmations encourage self-compassion, shifting focus from self-criticism to self-acknowledgment. Over time, this practice can cultivate a compassionate inner dialogue that supports healing and encourages resilience. Reframing thoughts through these positive lenses can significantly affect emotional well-being, making everyday challenges more manageable (A Beginner's Guide to Managing Pain Through Mindfulness, 2021).

Building community support is instrumental in managing chronic pain effectively. Engaging with support groups provides an invaluable platform for sharing experiences and developing coping strategies. These groups foster a sense of belonging and solidarity among members, reminding individuals that they are not alone in their journey. Participants find solace in shared stories, learning from each other's experiences and acquiring new methods to cope with their own pain. This connection alleviates feelings of isolation, boosting morale and encouraging emotional strength.

Social networks encompassing friends and family also play an important role in sustaining emotional resilience. Being able to lean on loved ones during tough times offers comfort and mitigates feelings of loneliness. Friends and family can provide both emotional support and practical advice, helping to navigate daily challenges associated with chronic pain. Whether it's offering a listening ear or participating in activities together, these connections enrich life beyond the limitations imposed by pain.

Community engagement extends beyond personal circles to broader social involvement. Participating in collective activities, whether online or in person, nurtures a sense of purpose and belonging. Individuals are encouraged to engage in interests and hobbies that bring joy, providing distraction from pain while enhancing life satisfaction. These activities not only provide pleasure but also cultivate a proactive approach to living, moving the focus away from pain towards meaningful engagement with others.

Mindfulness techniques for pain management offer structured approaches to integrating mindful practices into one's life seamlessly. Setting aside dedicated moments throughout the day for mindfulness exercises, such as meditation or breathing practices, ensures regular mental reprieve from pain. Encouraging habitual practices can create a consistent way to manage pain effectively, allowing individuals to build resilience steadily. This consistent practice reinforces the capacity to handle pain with calmness and strengthens one's ability to face challenging days with equanimity.

Future Mindfulness Goals

Creating a lifelong mindfulness plan is an essential step for individuals seeking lasting change in their lives, especially for those living with chronic pain. The journey towards integrating mindfulness into all life aspects requires consistency, patience, and the willingness to embrace growth through continuous practice and skill enhancement. This approach not only enriches daily experiences but also empowers individuals to navigate challenges with a renewed sense of calm and clarity.

To embark on this path, it's crucial to begin by crafting a personalized lifelong mindfulness plan. This plan serves as a roadmap, guiding your mindfulness journey with clear intentions and objectives. Think of it as an evolving document that adapts alongside you, reflecting new insights and achievements. By focusing on continuous practice, individuals can deepen their understanding of mindfulness techniques and enhance skills that promote mental and emotional resilience. A significant aspect of this process involves identifying specific areas where mindfulness can be most beneficial, such as pain management, stress reduction, or emotional regulation. Once these focus areas are pinpointed, setting realistic goals becomes more manageable, allowing for gradual and sustainable progress.

While crafting a mindfulness plan provides structure, engaging with continual learning resources further supports growth. Books, workshops, and online courses offer diverse perspectives and techniques that enrich one's mindfulness toolkit. For instance, attending workshops opens opportunities for interaction with experienced practitioners and fellow learners, fostering a sense of community and shared experience. Engaging with various resources helps to maintain motivation and inspires fresh approaches to incorporating mindfulness into everyday life.

It's equally important to recognize the power of setting measurable milestones within your mindfulness journey. These milestones act as benchmarks, enabling you to track progress and celebrate achievements, no matter how small they may seem. For example, beginning with the simple goal of meditating for five minutes each day sets a foundation upon which more extended practices can be built over time. Measuring progress instills a sense of accomplishment and reinforces commitment to ongoing practice and personal development. When goals are specific, measurable, achievable, relevant, and time-bound (SMART), they provide clear focus and direction, effectively steering efforts towards meaningful outcomes (<i>SMART Goals: The Health Coaching Cheat Code</i>, 2024).

Committing to mindfulness as a way of life promotes sustained transformation, nurturing a deeper connection with oneself and the surrounding world. This commitment goes beyond ticking off checkboxes; it's about cultivating a mindful state of being that permeates all aspects of life. Whether it's savoring the taste of food, appreciating the beauty of nature, or simply being present in conversations, mindfulness enriches these experiences by anchoring attention in the present moment. Over time, individuals discover that this mindful presence extends to challenging situations as well, allowing them to approach adversity with greater equanimity and resilience.

Moreover, adopting mindfulness as a lifelong commitment encourages a proactive stance toward personal growth. It fuels a mindset of curiosity and open-mindedness, inviting exploration of new ideas and concepts that challenge established patterns. This transformative journey not only enhances personal well-being but also positively influences relationships, communication, and overall quality of life. By embedding mindfulness into the fabric of daily existence, individuals can foster profound and lasting change that transcends the confines of any single book or resource.

For those seeking to integrate mindfulness more deeply into their lives, consider establishing regular reflection periods to review progress and reassess goals. Reflection allows for course correction when necessary, ensuring that the mindfulness plan remains aligned with evolving needs and aspirations. Taking time to reflect with honesty and kindness cultivates self-awareness and compassion, essential qualities for navigating life's ups and downs.

Bringing It All Together

The journey towards integrating mindfulness into everyday life represents a profound shift in how we interact with chronic pain. By embedding mindfulness into our routines, whether through mindful morning practices or simply pausing to breathe, we cultivate resilience and embrace a more harmonious existence. This chapter has illuminated the practical strategies to align daily actions with deeply-held values, empowering us to reshape our perspectives on challenges from impediments to opportunities for growth. The key lies in viewing pain not as an outsider but as a part of our experience that teaches us resilience and acceptance. Such a mindset allows us to engage actively with life despite the pain, fostering genuine connections with ourselves and others.

Looking ahead, the promise of lasting change through mindfulness hinges on commitment and continuous practice. By crafting a personalized lifelong mindfulness plan, individuals can create a roadmap tailored to their needs and aspirations. Setting specific, measurable goals and celebrating milestones along the way creates momentum, reinforcing a sense of achievement and perseverance. This dedicated approach cultivates a mindful state that enhances every aspect of life—from savoring simple moments to facing challenges with grace and strength. Embracing mindfulness is not just about momentary relief; it's about nurturing an enduring transformation that enriches our quality of life and empowers us to live authentically and purposefully amid chronic pain.

Reference List

Alis. (2025, January 21). *Emotional Coping Strategies for Chronic Pain - Alis Behavioral Health*. Alis Behavioral Health. https://www.alisbh.com/blog/emotional-coping-strategies-for-chronic-pain-23534/

Acceptance and Commitment therapy los angeles | ACT psychology. (2020). Cognitive Behavioral Therapy Los Angeles. https://cogbtherapy.com/acceptance-and-commitment-therapy-act-los-angeles

A Beginner's Guide to Managing Pain Through Mindfulness. (2021, November 23). Parkinson's Foundation. https://www.parkinson.org/blog/tips/pain-mindfulness

CIFI. (2024, August 26). *Acceptance and Commitment Therapy (ACT): Embracing Mindful Living for Personal Growth - Central Iowa Family Institute.* Central Iowa Family Institute. https://cif.institute/2024/08/26/acceptance-and-commitment-therapy-act-embracing-mindful-living-for-personal-growth/

How to integrate mindfulness into your everyday life. (2023, October 14). My Denver Therapy | Counseling in Denver, Colorado. https://mydenvertherapy.com/integrating-mindfulness-practices-into-everyday-life-for-improved-mental-health/

Microgility. (2024, October 30). *Realistic Mental Health Goals to Set in 2025.* Faith Behaviroal Health. https://faithbehavioralhealth.com/mental-health-goals/

SMART Goals: The Health Coaching Cheat Code. (2024, January 9). Functional Medicine Coaching Academy. https://functionalmedicinecoaching.org/blog/smart-goals/

What to Put on a Vision Board: Unlock Your Goals with These 10 Inspiring Ideas | AFFiNE. (2025). Affine.pro. https://affine.pro/blog/what-to-put-on-a-vision-board

Whitaker, A. (2023, November 9). *10 Simple Ways to Integrate Mindfulness into Your Daily Routine - SIYLI.* Siyli.org. https://siyli.org/resources/blog/10-simple-ways-to-integrate-mindfulness-into-your-daily-routine

https://www.briantracy.com/blog/author/brian-tracy. (2024, May 28). *Goal Setting for Success & Developing SMART Habits.* Brian Tracy.

https://www.briantracy.com/blog/personal-success/goal-setting/?srsltid=AfmBOoq9hR4CxFaXTC_Ehqp9UPKNO2E7id9H3Sc-IdQeYVTc2_ctBUXX

Conclusion

As we arrive at the end of our exploration into the role of mindfulness in managing chronic pain, let's take a moment to reflect on the journey we've embarked upon. This journey is not merely one of managing symptoms, but of transforming lives. For those living with chronic pain, mindfulness offers a beacon of hope — a means to alter the experience of pain and, perhaps more importantly, to reclaim parts of life that feel lost to suffering.

Imagine a life where the tight grip of chronic pain loosens, where you can engage more fully with the world around you. Mindfulness provides the tools needed to achieve this. Through simple yet powerful techniques such as mindful breathing, body scans, or meditation, you learn to notice pain without judgment, reducing its emotional impact. Many individuals report a significant decrease in their perception of pain when incorporating mindfulness into daily routines. The change isn't merely about hurting less but about feeling more alive, more connected.

Crucially, these practices don't happen in isolation. It's vital to recognize the immense value of community in the mindfulness journey. Pain can often make one feel isolated, trapped within a cycle that others might not understand. However, by joining group mindfulness sessions, you find solace in shared experiences and support. These groups foster a sense of belonging, reminding us that we are not alone in our struggles. Participating in a mindful community allows for mutual growth and understanding, helping reduce feelings of loneliness that so often accompany chronic conditions. Together, members inspire one another, sharing stories of resilience and breakthroughs that provide strength during difficult times.

Moreover, sustaining mindfulness as a lifelong practice promises continual benefits. Embracing mindfulness regularly enhances both mental and physical well-being. Over time, these practices become second nature, deeply ingrained in everyday life. Pain may still be present, but its control diminishes as your capacity for joy and satisfaction grows. By nurturing mindfulness, individuals report improvements not just in managing pain, but in overall life satisfaction, leading them to pursue passions and engage with loved ones more meaningfully. It becomes a cornerstone, supporting healthier lifestyles and promoting a fulfilling existence despite physical limitations.

A pivotal element of this transformation is learning to accept pain, not as an enemy to vanquish but as a part of the broader tapestry of life. Acceptance does not mean resignation; instead, it involves acknowledging pain's presence without letting it define you. When viewed through the lens of acceptance, pain loses its authority. It becomes a teacher rather than a tormentor. Responding with curiosity opens pathways to greater emotional resilience, allowing you to navigate challenges with flexibility and strength. It's about cultivating a mindset that welcomes growth, even from discomfort.

This journey is not one of quick fixes or miracle cures. Instead, it's about laying the foundation for profound and enduring change. As you integrate these practices into your life, remember that patience is key. Progress may be gradual, sometimes imperceptible, but every step taken toward self-awareness and self-compassion represents victory over despair. Celebrate these small triumphs as they accumulate into significant transformations.

In closing, let us reaffirm the central message of our journey together: embracing mindfulness offers a transformative approach to managing chronic pain, enhancing life richly and profoundly. You have discovered how mindfulness empowers you to reshape the narrative of pain, enabling you to live with greater intention, resilience, and fulfillment. Remember, the pursuit of wellness is personal and continuous—one filled with opportunities to learn, adapt, and thrive.

As you move forward, take with you the knowledge that pain does not dictate your story. You possess the power to redefine your relationship with it, crafting a future where mindfulness illuminates each new day. Let the practices outlined in this book guide you toward a path of healing and hope. May your journey be filled with compassion—for yourself, for others, and for the world you inhabit.

About the Authors:
The Æthereal Dreams Collective

This book is the collaborative work of the **Æthereal Dreams Collective**, a diverse group of authors united by their shared passion for mindfulness, holistic healing, and the transformative power of self-discovery. Each member of the collective brings a unique blend of professional expertise, creative insight, and personal experience to the table, making this book a rich tapestry of knowledge and empathy.

Diverse Professional Backgrounds

The authors of the Æthereal Dreams Collective come from a wide range of disciplines, including:

Medicine: Practitioners with years of experience in pain management, neurology, and integrative health, offering evidence-based insights into the science of mindfulness and its impact on chronic pain.

Art and Design: Creative minds who infuse the book with visually engaging content, such as illustrations, diagrams, and meditative visualizations, making complex concepts accessible and inspiring.

Life Sciences: Experts in psychology, neuroscience, and biology, who provide a deep understanding of the mind-body connection and the physiological mechanisms behind pain and healing.

Personal Life Experiences

Beyond their professional credentials, the authors of the Æthereal Dreams Collective have lived experiences that bring authenticity and depth to their writing. Many have faced their own battles with chronic pain, emotional trauma, or mental health challenges, and have discovered mindfulness as a powerful tool for healing and transformation. These personal journeys allow them to write with **empathy, compassion, and a genuine understanding** of what it means to live with pain and seek relief.

A Collaborative Vision

The Æthereal Dreams Collective was born out of a shared belief in the power of collaboration and the importance of addressing pain management from multiple perspectives. By combining their diverse expertise and personal stories, the authors have created a book that is both **practical and deeply human**, offering readers not only tools for pain relief but also a sense of connection and hope.

Mission and Purpose

The collective's mission is to empower individuals to take control of their pain and their lives through mindfulness, self-compassion, and holistic healing. They believe that pain, while challenging, can also be a catalyst for growth, self-discovery, and transformation. Through this book, they aim to inspire readers to embrace mindfulness as a way of life, fostering resilience, emotional well-being, and a renewed sense of purpose.

Why This Book Matters

The Æthereal Dreams Collective understands that chronic pain is not just a physical experience but a deeply emotional and psychological one. Their goal is to provide readers with a **comprehensive, accessible, and**

compassionate guide to mindfulness for pain management—one that addresses the whole person, not just their symptoms. By sharing their knowledge, experiences, and practical tools, the authors hope to help readers find relief, build resilience, and reclaim their lives.

Final Thought for Jean-François:

To our beloved son, Jean-François, who has faced the relentless challenge of chronic pain with unwavering courage and grace for nearly four years, this book is a testament to the strength and resilience you embody. Your journey has been a profound inspiration to us and to all who know you. Though the beast of pain may linger, we hope these pages offer you solace, tools, and a reminder that you are never alone. We are here, always, walking beside you, holding your hand through every moment of struggle and triumph. May you find moments of calm and serenity amidst the storm, and may your spirit continue to shine brightly, illuminating the path for others who walk a similar road. You are our heart, our hope, and our greatest inspiration. With all our love, always. —Marie José and Pierre

Glossary

Acceptance – A core principle of mindfulness that involves acknowledging pain without resistance or judgment, helping to reduce emotional suffering.

Acute Pain – Short-term pain that occurs due to injury, surgery, or illness, usually resolving once the underlying cause is treated.

Affirmations – Positive statements or self-talk used in mindfulness practice to cultivate resilience and emotional well-being.

Awareness – A state of conscious perception that is a key component of mindfulness, allowing individuals to observe sensations, thoughts, and emotions without attachment.

Body Scan Meditation – A mindfulness practice where attention is directed systematically through different parts of the body to increase awareness and reduce tension.

Breathwork – The practice of controlled breathing techniques that help regulate the nervous system and reduce pain-related stress.

Catastrophizing – A cognitive distortion where individuals exaggerate the perceived severity of their pain, often leading to increased distress and suffering.

Chronic Pain – Persistent pain lasting more than three months, often without a clear physical cause, impacting daily life and emotional health.

Compassionate Self-Talk – The practice of using kind and supportive language when addressing oneself, reducing negative self-judgment related to chronic pain.

Complementary Therapies – Non-medical treatments such as mindfulness, acupuncture, and yoga used alongside traditional medicine for pain management.

Default Mode Network (DMN) – A set of interconnected brain regions active during self-referential thinking; mindfulness reduces DMN activity, decreasing ruminative thoughts about pain.

Diaphragmatic Breathing – A deep-breathing technique that activates the parasympathetic nervous system, promoting relaxation and reducing pain intensity.

Distraction Technique – A mindfulness strategy where individuals redirect attention away from pain to lessen its perceived intensity.

Emotional Regulation – The ability to manage and respond to emotional experiences effectively, often improved through mindfulness practices.

Empirical Research – Scientific studies that provide evidence for the effectiveness of mindfulness in reducing chronic pain and stress.

Endorphins – Natural pain-relieving chemicals produced by the body, which mindfulness and meditation can help stimulate.

Focused Attention Meditation – A form of mindfulness where individuals concentrate on a specific sensation, such as breath or sound, to anchor awareness and reduce pain-related distress.

Fibromyalgia – A chronic pain disorder characterized by widespread musculoskeletal pain, fatigue, and cognitive difficulties, often managed with mindfulness-based techniques.

Functional MRI (fMRI) – A brain imaging technique used in research to show how mindfulness alters neural activity related to pain perception.

Guided Imagery – A mindfulness technique that involves visualizing calming or pleasant scenes to shift attention away from pain and promote relaxation.

Grounding Techniques – Strategies used in mindfulness to bring awareness to the present moment and reduce pain-related anxiety.

Holistic Healing – A comprehensive approach to health that considers the mind, body, and spirit, integrating mindfulness with traditional medical treatments.

Hyperalgesia – An increased sensitivity to pain, often exacerbated by stress and emotional distress, which mindfulness practices can help mitigate.

Interoception – The awareness of internal bodily sensations, which mindfulness enhances to improve pain management.

Intentional Awareness – The act of purposefully focusing on the present moment to cultivate mindfulness and reduce pain intensity.

Integration with Medical Treatment – The practice of combining mindfulness with conventional medical approaches for a balanced pain management strategy.

Journaling for Mindfulness – A reflective practice where individuals document their pain experiences, emotions, and progress to increase self-awareness and resilience.

Judgment-Free Awareness – A mindfulness principle that encourages observing thoughts and sensations without labeling them as good or bad.

Kindness-Based Meditation – A mindfulness technique focused on cultivating compassion toward oneself and others, reducing stress and emotional suffering related to pain.

Longitudinal Studies – Research that follows participants over an extended period to assess the long-term effects of mindfulness on chronic pain.

Meditation – A practice of focused attention and awareness, often used in mindfulness-based pain management programs.

Mind-Body Connection – The relationship between mental states and physical health, a key concept in mindfulness-based pain management.

Mindful Acceptance – The practice of acknowledging pain and discomfort without trying to change or resist it.

Mindfulness-Based Stress Reduction (MBSR) – A structured eight-week program developed by Dr. Jon Kabat-Zinn to help individuals manage chronic pain and stress.

Mobility Adaptations – Adjustments in mindfulness exercises to accommodate individuals with limited movement due to chronic pain conditions.

Neuroplasticity – The brain's ability to reorganize and form new neural connections, which mindfulness practices can enhance to reduce chronic pain.

Neuropathic Pain – Pain caused by nerve damage or dysfunction, which mindfulness can help manage by altering the perception of discomfort.

Non-Striving – A mindfulness principle emphasizing being present without the need to achieve a specific outcome, fostering a relaxed approach to pain management.

Opioid System Modulation – The process by which mindfulness influences natural pain-relief mechanisms in the body, potentially reducing reliance on medications.

Observational Awareness – The act of neutrally observing bodily sensations, thoughts, and emotions without reacting to them.

Pain Reframing – A cognitive technique used in mindfulness to shift how pain is perceived, reducing distress and emotional suffering.

Parasympathetic Nervous System – The part of the autonomic nervous system responsible for relaxation and healing, activated through mindfulness and breathwork.

Progressive Muscle Relaxation – A mindfulness technique that involves tensing and releasing muscles to promote relaxation and pain relief.

Psychogenic Pain – Pain influenced by psychological factors such as stress and emotions, often addressed through mindfulness-based cognitive techniques.

Quality of Life Improvement – The enhancement of overall well-being through mindfulness practices that help manage chronic pain effectively.

Quieting the Mind – A mindfulness skill that reduces mental chatter and stress, leading to decreased pain perception.

Radical Acceptance – A mindfulness practice that encourages complete acknowledgment of pain and suffering without resistance, fostering emotional resilience.

Rumination – Repetitive negative thinking about pain or distress, which mindfulness techniques help to break.

Self-Compassion – The practice of treating oneself with kindness and understanding, a key component in mindfulness for pain management.

Sensory Awareness – The heightened perception of bodily sensations through mindfulness, allowing individuals to notice and manage pain more effectively.

Somatic Mindfulness – A practice focused on bodily sensations to increase awareness and reduce pain-related stress.

Stress Response – The body's reaction to perceived threats, which mindfulness helps regulate to prevent pain flare-ups.

Tailored Mindfulness Practices – Adjusting mindfulness techniques to fit individual pain conditions, ensuring accessibility and effectiveness.

Thought Labeling – A mindfulness technique where individuals categorize their thoughts to reduce their emotional impact.

Trigger Awareness – The recognition of environmental or emotional factors that worsen pain, allowing for proactive mindfulness-based coping strategies.

Uncertainty Tolerance – The ability to accept unpredictability in pain experiences, a skill enhanced through mindfulness.

Unraveling Cognitive Patterns – The mindfulness-based approach of identifying and modifying negative thought loops related to pain.

Visualization Techniques – Mindfulness exercises that use mental imagery to create a sense of calm and reduce pain perception.

Vagus Nerve Activation – Stimulation of the vagus nerve through mindfulness and breathwork, promoting relaxation and decreasing pain intensity.

Walking Meditation – A mindfulness practice that involves focusing on the sensations of movement, often used for those who find seated meditation uncomfortable.

Well-Being Metrics – The indicators of emotional and physical health improvements due to mindfulness-based pain management.

X-Factor of Mindfulness – The unique ability of mindfulness to transform the perception of pain without requiring external interventions.

Yoga for Chronic Pain – A form of mindful movement that integrates breath awareness and gentle stretching to alleviate pain.

Zen Mindset – A mindfulness approach that encourages simplicity, non-attachment, and present-moment focus for pain relief.

References

1. 10 Types of Moving Meditations—Benefits of Mindful Movement | The Buddhist Center. (n.d.). Tnlsf.org. https://tnlsf.org/10-types-of-moving-meditations-benefits-of-mindful-movement/

2. A Beginner's Guide to Managing Pain Through Mindfulness. (2021, November 23). Parkinson's Foundation. https://www.parkinson.org/blog/tips/pain-mindfulness

3. Ainsworth, B., Atkinson, M. J., Eman AlBedah, Duncan, S., Groot, J., Jacobsen, P., James, A., Jenkins, T., Katerina Kylisova, Marks, E., Osborne, E. L., Masha Remskar, & Underhill, R. (2023, May 20). Current Tensions and Challenges in Mindfulness Research and Practice. https://doi.org/10.1007/s10879-023-09584-9

4. Alis. (2025, January 21). Emotional Coping Strategies for Chronic Pain - Alis Behavioral Health. Alis Behavioral Health. https://www.alisbh.com/blog/emotional-coping-strategies-for-chronic-pain-23534/

5. AlSubaie, Aeishaa AlSubaie, Bajawi, Zahra Awaji, Hassan, A., Shabani, K. M., Ibrahim, S. A., Nasser, A., Owaid, M., Khalaf, H., Alhamadan, Fahad Hamadan, Al-Qahtani, Atef Fahid Ayed, Aldhafeeri, Tahani Huwaydi, Aldhafeeri, Mashael Huwaydi, Abdullah, A. I., Mubarak, A.-S. N., & Mohammed. (2024, December). Integrating Mindfulness-Based Interventions into Mental Health Nursing: A Review of Evidence, Biochemical Mechanisms, and Implementation Challenges. Journal of Medicinal and Chemical Sciences; Sami Publishing Company (SPC). https://doi.org/10.26655/JMCHEMSCI.2024.12.8

6. American Cancer Society. (2020, December 2). Practice Mindfulness and Relaxation. Www.cancer.org. https://www.cancer.org/cancer/survivorship/coping/practice-mindfulness-and-relaxation.html

7. Ankrom, S. (2024, February 16). Need a Breather? Try These 9 Breathing Exercises to Relieve Anxiety. Verywell Mind. https://www.verywellmind.com/abdominal-breathing-2584115

8. Author, S. development. (2023, May 18). Unearthing the Secret to Amplified Personal Growth: Collective Mindfulness. Medium. https://medium.com/@yacuncao2/unearthing-the-secret-to-amplified-personal-growth-collective-mindfulness-61595f0779bc

9. Bansal, M. (2020, January 30). Encouraging Mindfulness Through Design - Mihika Bansal - Medium. Medium. https://mihikabansal.medium.com/encouraging-mindfulness-through-design-7e7465235830

10. Banerjee, M., Cavanagh, K., & Strauss, C. (2017, November 6). Barriers to Mindfulness: a Path Analytic Model Exploring the Role of Rumination and Worry in Predicting Psychological and Physical Engagement in an Online Mindfulness-Based Intervention. Mindfulness. https://doi.org/10.1007/s12671-017-0837-4

11. Benefits of Guided Imagery for Pain Management | Beaumont | Beaumont Health. (n.d.). Www.beaumont.org. https://www.beaumont.org/services/pain-management-services/benefits-of-guided-imagery-for-pain-management

12. Bentley, T. G. K., D'Andrea-Penna, G., Rakic, M., Arce, N., LaFaille, M., Berman, R., Cooley, K., & Sprimont, P. (2023, November 21). Breathing Practices for Stress and Anxiety Reduction: Conceptual Framework of Implementation

Guidelines Based on a Systematic Review of the Published Literature. Brain Sciences. https://doi.org/10.3390/brainsci13121612

13. Calderone, A., Latella, D., Impellizzeri, F., Pasquale, P. de, Famà, F., Quartarone, A., & Calabrò, R. S. (2024, November 15). Neurobiological Changes Induced by Mindfulness and Meditation: A Systematic Review. Biomedicines; Multidisciplinary Digital Publishing Institute. https://doi.org/10.3390/biomedicines12112613

14. Calligraphy, A. (2024, November 28). Spiritual Mindfulness: Everyday Chores as a Path to Presence. Medium; ILLUMINATION. https://medium.com/illumination/spiritual-mindfulness-everyday-chores-as-a-path-to-presence-cd2c246f4954

15. CIFI. (2024, August 26). Acceptance and Commitment Therapy (ACT): Embracing Mindful Living for Personal Growth - Central Iowa Family Institute. Central Iowa Family Institute. https://cif.institute/2024/08/26/acceptance-and-commitment-therapy-act-embracing-mindful-living-for-personal-growth/

16. Change, I. (2021, August 24). How to Overcome Obstacles to Mindfulness. Intelligent Change. https://www.intelligentchange.com/blogs/read/how-to-overcome-obstacles-to-mindfulness?srsltid=AfmBOorFlOmw9KN_Umow4gbnn-l1OMsfC5q6NR6QG07oJCZefLFHylzN

17. Charness, G., Le Bihan, Y., & Villeval, M. C. (2024, January 1). Mindfulness training, cognitive performance and stress reduction. Journal of Economic Behavior & Organization. https://doi.org/10.1016/j.jebo.2023.10.027

18.   Cherpak, C. E. (2019, August). Mindful Eating: A Review Of How The Stress-Digestion-Mindfulness Triad May Modulate And Improve Gastrointestinal And Digestive Function. Integrative Medicine: A Clinician's Journal. https://pmc.ncbi.nlm.nih.gov/articles/PMC7219460/

19.   Cohen, S. P., Wang, E. J., Doshi, T. L., Vase, L., Cawcutt, K. A., & Tontisirin, N. (2022, March). Chronic pain and infection: mechanisms, causes, conditions, treatments, and controversies. BMJ Medicine. https://doi.org/10.1136/bmjmed-2021-000108

20.   Cosio, D., & Sujata Swaroop. (2016, March 30). The Use of Mind-body Medicine in Chronic Pain Management: Differential Trends and Session-by-Session Changes in Anxiety. Journal of Pain Management & Medicine. https://pmc.ncbi.nlm.nih.gov/articles/PMC4855874/

21.   Crego, A., Yela, J. R., Gómez-Martínez, M. Á., Riesco-Matías, P., & Petisco-Rodríguez, C. (2021, January 21). Relationships between Mindfulness, Purpose in Life, Happiness, Anxiety, and Depression: Testing a Mediation Model in a Sample of Women. International Journal of Environmental Research and Public Health. https://doi.org/10.3390/ijerph18030925

22.   CST (she/her), K. E., LCSW, PMH-C. (2023, October 18). Care Coordination: The Benefits of Collaborative Healthcare. Wildflower Center for Emotional Health. https://www.wildflowerllc.com/care-coordination-the-benefits-of-collaborative-healthcare/

23.   Deschene, L. (2010, July 28). Mindfulness in Everyday Tasks: How to Get the Most from Your Chores. Tiny Buddha.

https://tinybuddha.com/blog/mindfulness-in-everyday-tasks-5-ways-chores-can-make-you-happier/

24.   Dr. Kirilyuk Inna Anatolyivna. (2023, April 3). The Many Benefits Of Meditation and Mindfulness For Seniors. Megawecare; Mega We Care. https://www.megawecare.com/good-health-by-yourself/healthy-aging/meditation-for-seniors

25.   Duenas, M., Ojeda, B., Salazar, A., Mico, J. A., & Failde, I. (2016, June). A review of chronic pain impact on patients, their social environment and the health care system. Journal of Pain Research. https://doi.org/10.2147/JPR.S105892

26.   Dubey, A., & Muley, P. A. (2023, November 22). Meditation: A Promising Approach for Alleviating Chronic Pain. Cureus. https://doi.org/10.7759/cureus.49244

27.   Egel, K. (2024, December 4). Kim Egel. Kim Egel. https://www.kimegel.com/blog/2024/12/4/mental-health-benefits-of-journaling-gaining-mindfulness-via-a-journaling-practice

28.   Elendu, C. (2024, July 12). The evolution of ancient healing practices: From shamanism to Hippocratic medicine: A review. Medicine. https://doi.org/10.1097/MD.0000000000039005

29.   Farr, M., Brant, H., Patel, R., Linton, M.-J., Ambler, N., Vyas, S., Wedge, H., Watkins, S., & Horwood, J. (2021, June 28). Experiences of Patient-Led Chronic Pain Peer Support Groups After Pain Management Programs: A Qualitative Study. Pain Medicine. https://doi.org/10.1093/pm/pnab189

30.   Five Healthy Coping Skills For Facing Setbacks | BetterHelp. (n.d.). Www.betterhelp.com.

https://www.betterhelp.com/advice/mindfulness/five-healthy-coping-skills-for-facing-setbacks/

31.   Forgeron, P. A., King, S., Stinson, J. N., McGrath, P. J., MacDonald, A. J., & Chambers, C. T. (2010). Social functioning and peer relationships in children and adolescents with chronic pain: A systematic review. Pain Research & Management; Pulsus Group Inc. https://doi.org/10.1155/2010/820407

32.   Franqueiro, A. R., Yoon, J., Crago, M. A., Curiel, M., & Wilson, J. M. (2023, October 27). The Interconnection Between Social Support and Emotional Distress Among Individuals with Chronic Pain: A Narrative Review. Psychology Research and Behavior Management. https://doi.org/10.2147/PRBM.S410606

33.   Fritz, J. M., Rhon, D. I., Garland, E. L., Hanley, A. W., Greenlee, T. A., Fino, N. F., Martin, B. I., Highland, K. B., & Greene, T. (2022, September 7). The Effectiveness of a Mindfulness-Based Intervention Integrated with Physical Therapy (MIND-PT) for Post-Surgical Rehabilitation after Lumbar Surgery: A Protocol for a Randomized Controlled Trial as Part of the Back Pain Consortium (BACPAC) Research Program. https://doi.org/10.1093/pm/pnac138

34.   Gaylord, S. A., Palsson, O. S., Garland, E. L., Faurot, K. R., Coble, R. S., Mann, D. J., Frey, W., Leniek, K., & Whitehead, W. E. (2011, September). Mindfulness Training Reduces the Severity of Irritable Bowel Syndrome in Women: Results of a Randomized Controlled Trial. American Journal of Gastroenterology. https://doi.org/10.1038/ajg.2011.184

35.   Givler, A., & Maani-Fogelman, P. A. (2023). The importance of cultural competence in pain and palliative care. National Library of Medicine; StatPearls Publishing. https://www.ncbi.nlm.nih.gov/books/NBK493154/

36. Gotter, A. (2018, April 20). What Is the 4-7-8 Breathing Technique? Healthline; Healthline Media. https://www.healthline.com/health/4-7-8-breathing

37. Grant. (2022, March 29). Dr. Daya Grant. Dr. Daya Grant. https://www.dayagrant.com/blog/a-mindful-strategy-for-facing-setbacks

38. Hardison, M. E., & Roll, S. C. (2016, April 1). Mindfulness Interventions in Physical Rehabilitation: A Scoping Review. American Journal of Occupational Therapy. https://doi.org/10.5014/ajot.2016.018069

39. Harris, K., Jackson, J. L., Webster, H. L., Farrow, J. A., Zhao, Y., & Hohmann, L. (2023, September 21). Mindfulness-Based Stress Reduction (MBSR) for Chronic Pain Management in the Community Pharmacy Setting: A Cross-Sectional Survey of the General Public's Knowledge and Perceptions. Pharmacy; Multidisciplinary Digital Publishing Institute. https://doi.org/10.3390/pharmacy11050150

40. Harvard Health Publishing. (2022, May 24). The health benefits of tai chi. Harvard Health; Harvard Health. https://www.health.harvard.edu/staying-healthy/the-health-benefits-of-tai-chi

41. Hilton, L., Hempel, S., Ewing, B. A., Apaydin, E., Xenakis, L., Newberry, S., Colaiaco, B., Maher, A. R., Shanman, R. M., Sorbero, M. E., & Maglione, M. A. (2017, September 22). Mindfulness meditation for chronic pain: Systematic review and meta-analysis. Annals of Behavioral Medicine. https://doi.org/10.1007/s12160-016-9844-2

42. History of MBSR. (n.d.). MBSR Collaborative. https://mbsrcollaborative.com/history-of-mbsr

43.   Hofmann, S. G., & Gómez, A. F. (2018). Mindfulness-Based Interventions for Anxiety and Depression. Psychiatric Clinics of North America. https://doi.org/10.1016/j.psc.2017.08.008

44.   Home. (n.d.). Mindfulness Based Stress Reduction. https://mbsrtraining.com/

45.   How Home Health Care Professionals Address Chronic Pain. (2025). Regencyhcs.com. https://www.regencyhcs.com/blog/how-home-health-care-professionals-address-chronic-pain?25b4f686_page=5

46.   How to create a supportive environment for residents with chronic pain. (2025). Downersgrovehc.com. https://www.downersgrovehc.com/blog/how-to-create-a-supportive-environment-for-residents-with-chronic-pain?372b7fa3_page=3

47.   How to integrate mindfulness into your everyday life. (2023, October 14). My Denver Therapy | Counseling in Denver, Colorado. https://mydenvertherapy.com/integrating-mindfulness-practices-into-everyday-life-for-improved-mental-health/

48.   How. (2024, August 5). Calm Blog. Calm Blog. https://www.calm.com/blog/meditation-room-ideas

49.   Ikigai Transformations- Live on Purpose. (2024). Apple Podcasts. https://podcasts.apple.com/pe/podcast/ikigai-transfromations-live-on-purpose/id1591691354

50.   Innis, A. D., Tolea, M. I., & Galvin, J. E. (2021, January 1). The Effect of Baseline Patient and Caregiver Mindfulness on Dementia Outcomes. Journal of Alzheimer's Disease. https://doi.org/10.3233/JAD-201292

51.   jason. (2024, October 23). 5 Mindful Movement Practices for Optimal Health and Well-Being - Health & Wellness Canada. Health & Wellness Canada. https://www.healthcouncilcanada.ca/5-mindful-movement-practices-for-optimal-health-and-well-being/

52.   Joo, J. H., Bone, L., Forte, J., Kirley, E., Lynch, T., & Aboumatar, H. (2022). The benefits and challenges of established peer support programmes for patients, informal caregivers, and healthcare providers. Family Practice. https://doi.org/10.1093/fampra/cmac004

53.   Katz, J., Rosenbloom, B. N., & Fashler, S. (2015, April). Chronic Pain, Psychopathology, and DSM-5 Somatic Symptom Disorder. The Canadian Journal of Psychiatry. https://doi.org/10.1177/070674371506000402

54.   Keng, S. L., Smoski, M. J., & Robins, C. J. (2011). Effects of Mindfulness on Psychological health: a Review of Empirical Studies. Clinical Psychology Review. https://doi.org/10.1016/j.cpr.2011.04.006

55.   Koithan, M., & Farrell, C. (2010, June 1). Indigenous Native American Healing Traditions. The Journal for Nurse Practitioners; National Library of Medicine. https://doi.org/10.1016/j.nurpra.2010.03.016

56.   Kriakous, S. A., Elliott, K. A., Lamers, C., & Owen, R. (2021, September 24). The effectiveness of mindfulness-based stress reduction on the psychological functioning of healthcare professionals: A systematic review. Mindfulness. https://doi.org/10.1007/s12671-020-01500-9

57.   Lee, C. (2024, April 24). Healing Ourselves as Indigenous People. Www.aft.org. https://www.aft.org/hc/spring2024/lee

58. Li, X., Ma, L., & Li, Q. (2022, June 30). How Mindfulness Affects Life Satisfaction: Based on the Mindfulness-to-Meaning Theory. Frontiers in Psychology. https://doi.org/10.3389/fpsyg.2022.887940

59. Lindsay, E. K., Young, S., Brown, K. W., Smyth, J. M., & Creswell, J. D. (2019, February 11). Mindfulness training reduces loneliness and increases social contact in a randomized controlled trial. Proceedings of the National Academy of Sciences. https://doi.org/10.1073/pnas.1813588116

60. Lu, C., Moliadze, V., & Nees, F. (2023, November 9). Dynamic processes of mindfulness-based alterations in pain perception. Frontiers in Neuroscience; Frontiers Media. https://doi.org/10.3389/fnins.2023.1253559

61. Madeson, M. (2022, October 27). Mindfulness in counseling: 8 best techniques & interventions. PositivePsychology.com. https://positivepsychology.com/mindfulness-in-counseling/

62. Main Section | Community Tool Box. (2025). Ku.edu. http://ctb.ku.edu/en/table-of-contents/spirituality-and-community-building/mindfulness-community-building/main

63. Marano, S. (2023, July 10). Pathway to Growth - How Personal Growth Will Change Your Life. LSC. https://www.lavenderskycounselling.com/post/personal-growth-how-personal-growth-will-change-your-life

64. Mayo Clinic Staff. (2022, October 11). Mindfulness exercises. Mayo Clinic. https://www.mayoclinic.org/healthy-lifestyle/consumer-health/in-depth/mindfulness-exercises/art-20046356

65.   Mayo Clinic. (2023, December 14). Meditation: A simple, fast way to reduce stress. Mayo Clinic. https://www.mayoclinic.org/tests-procedures/meditation/in-depth/meditation/art-20045858

66.   Mead, E. (2019, June). What is Mindful Self-Compassion? (Incl. Exercises + Workbooks). PositivePsychology.com. https://positivepsychology.com/mindful-self-compassion/

67.   Meditative Journey: Storytelling in Guided Meditation. (2023). Themindorchestra.com. https://www.themindorchestra.com/blog/meditative-guided-meditation-storytelling

68.   Mental Health Foundation. (2022). How to look after your mental health using mindfulness. Www.mentalhealth.org.uk. https://www.mentalhealth.org.uk/explore-mental-health/publications/how-look-after-your-mental-health-using-mindfulness

69.   Microgility. (2024, October 30). Realistic Mental Health Goals to Set in 2025. Faith Behaviroal Health. https://faithbehavioralhealth.com/mental-health-goals/

70.   Mindfulness for Fibromyalgia. (2022, May 13). Breathworks. https://www.breathworks-mindfulness.org.uk/blog/mindfulness-for-fibromyalgia

71.   Mindfulness Mentoring | The Mindfulness Network. (2020, July 2). The Mindfulness Network | Serving the Community through Mindfulness-Based Supervision, Retreats and Training Courses. http://home.mindfulness-network.org/practice-mindfulness/mindfulness-mentoring/

72. Mindfulness Techniques For Pain Management. (n.d.). Physiopedia. https://www.physio-pedia.com/Mindfulness_Techniques_For_Pain_Management

73. Mindfulness-based stress reduction (MBSR) - MBSR exercises. (n.d.). Guy's and St Thomas' NHS Foundation Trust. https://www.guysandstthomas.nhs.uk/health-information/mindfulness-based-stress-reduction-mbsr/mbsr-exercises

74. Namjoo, S., Borjali, A., Seirafi, M., & Assarzadegan, F. (2019, October 20). Use of Mindfulness-based Cognitive Therapy to Change Pain-related Cognitive Processing in Patients with Primary Headache: A Randomized Trial with Attention Placebo Control Group. Anesthesiology and Pain Medicine. https://doi.org/10.5812/aapm.91927

75. Neff, K. (2024). Self-compassion practices. Self-Compassion. https://self-compassion.org/self-compassion-practices/

76. New. (2021). Deep Mindfulness. Deep Mindfulness. https://deepmindfulness.io/mentorship

77. Niazi, A. K., & Niazi, S. K. (2011). Mindfulness-based Stress reduction: a non-pharmacological Approach for Chronic Illnesses. North American Journal of Medical Sciences. https://doi.org/10.4297/najms.2011.320

78. Oh, V. K. S., Sarwar, A., & Pervez, N. (2022, December 21). The study of mindfulness as an intervening factor for enhanced psychological well-being in building the level of resilience. Figshare.com. https://doi.org/10.3389/fpsyg.2022.1056834

79.   Pal, P., Hauck, C., Goldstein, E., Bobinet, K., & Bradley, C. (2018, December 13). 5 simple mindfulness practices for daily life. Mindful. https://www.mindful.org/take-a-mindful-moment-5-simple-practices-for-daily-life/

80.   Puterman, E., & Epel, E. (2012, November). An Intricate Dance: Life Experience, Multisystem Resiliency, and Rate of Telomere Decline Throughout the Lifespan. Social and Personality Psychology Compass. https://doi.org/10.1111/j.1751-9004.2012.00465.x

81.   Raypole, C. (2020, March 26). Body Scan Meditation: Benefits and How to Do It. Healthline. https://www.healthline.com/health/body-scan-meditation

82.   Riopel, L. (2019, April 10). Goal Setting in Counseling and Therapy (Incl. Workbooks & Templates). PositivePsychology.com. https://positivepsychology.com/goal-setting-counseling-therapy/

83.   Rose, M. (2024, June 10). Self-help Strategies: Rose Behavioral Health's Guide to Personal Wellness - Rose Behavioral Health. Rose Behavioral Health. https://www.rosebehavioralhealth.com/self-help-strategies-rose-behavioral-healths-guide-to-personal-wellness/

84.   Rosen, M. A. (2019). Teamwork in healthcare: Key discoveries enabling safer, high-quality care. American Psychologist; NCBI. https://doi.org/10.1037/amp0000298

85.   Roth, I., Tiedt, M., Miller, V., Barnhill, J., Chilcoat, A., Gardiner, P., Faurot, K., Karvelas, K., Busby, K., Gaylord, S., & Leeman, J. (2023, September 27). Integrative medical group visits for patients with chronic pain: results of a pilot single-site hybrid implementation-effectiveness feasibility study. Frontiers in Pain Research. https://doi.org/10.3389/fpain.2023.1147588

86.   Rusch, H. L., Rosario, M., Levison, L. M., Olivera, A., Livingston, W. S., Wu, T., & Gill, J. M. (2018, December 21). The effect of mindfulness meditation on sleep quality: a systematic review and meta-analysis of randomized controlled trials. Annals of the New York Academy of Sciences. https://doi.org/10.1111/nyas.13996

87.   Sani, N. A., Yusoff, S. S. M., Norhayati, M. N., & Zainudin, A. M. (2023, February 5). Tai Chi Exercise for Mental and Physical Well-Being in Patients with Depressive Symptoms: A Systematic Review and Meta-Analysis. International Journal of Environmental Research and Public Health. https://doi.org/10.3390/ijerph20042828

88.   Schuman-Olivier, Z., Trombka, M., Lovas, D. A., Brewer, J. A., Vago, D. R., Gawande, R., Dunne, J. P., Lazar, S. W., Loucks, E. B., & Fulwiler, C. (2020). Mindfulness and behavior change. Harvard Review of Psychiatry. https://doi.org/10.1097/HRP.0000000000000277

89.   Scott, E. (2024, February 12). What is body scan meditation? Verywell Mind. https://www.verywellmind.com/body-scan-meditation-why-and-how-3144782

90.   Senior Lifestyle. (2025, February 11). Mindfulness for Caregivers: Cultivating Presence and Resilience in Daily Life. Senior Lifestyle. https://www.seniorlifestyle.com/resources/blog/mindfulness-for-caregivers-cultivating-presence-and-resilience-in-daily-life/

91.   Sheikhrabori, A., Peyrovi, H., & Khankeh, H. (2022, February 15). The Main Features of Resilience in Healthcare Providers: A Scoping Review. Medical Journal of the Islamic Republic of Iran. https://doi.org/10.47176/mjiri.36.3

92.   Shlafman, M. (2023, June 2). Origins Holistic Psychotherapy | Dr. Michelle Shlafman LPC, ACS. Origins Holistic Psychotherapy | Dr. Michelle Shlafman LPC, ACS. https://michelleshlafman.com/blog/empowering-yourself-to-heal-mindfulness-and-self-compassion-for-chronic-pain

93.   SMART Goals: The Health Coaching Cheat Code. (2024, January 9). Functional Medicine Coaching Academy. https://functionalmedicinecoaching.org/blog/smart-goals/

94.   Sodeman, L. (2020, September 25). Use mindfulness to cope with chronic pain. Www.mayoclinichealthsystem.org. https://www.mayoclinichealthsystem.org/hometown-health/speaking-of-health/use-mindfulness-to-cope-with-chronic-pain

95.   Srour, R. A., & Keyes, D. (2024). Lifestyle Mindfulness In Clinical Practice. PubMed; StatPearls Publishing. https://www.ncbi.nlm.nih.gov/books/NBK599498/

96.   Stange, K. C., Etz, R. S., Gullett, H., Sweeney, S. A., Miller, W. L., Jaén, C. R., Crabtree, B. F., Nutting, P. A., & Glasgow, R. E. (2014, March 18). Metrics for Assessing Improvements in Primary Health Care. Annual Review of Public Health. https://doi.org/10.1146/annurev-publhealth-032013-182438

97.   Sturgeon, J. A., & Zautra, A. J. (2010, March 2). Resilience: A New Paradigm for Adaptation to Chronic Pain. Current Pain and Headache Reports. https://doi.org/10.1007/s11916-010-0095-9

98.   Sturgeon, J. A., & Zautra, A. J. (2013, January 22). Psychological Resilience, Pain Catastrophizing, and Positive Emotions: Perspectives on Comprehensive Modeling of

Individual Pain Adaptation. Current Pain and Headache Reports. https://doi.org/10.1007/s11916-012-0317-4

99.   Sutton, J. (2020, July 24). Practicing Mindfulness in Groups: 9 Activities and Exercises. PositivePsychology.com. https://positivepsychology.com/group-mindfulness-activities/

100.   Tabish, S. A. (2008). Complementary and Alternative Healthcare: Is it Evidence-based? International Journal of Health Sciences. https://pmc.ncbi.nlm.nih.gov/articles/PMC3068720/

101.   Team, B. E. (2024, March 4). Boost Energy Levels With The Mind-Body Connection | BetterHelp. Betterhelp.com; BetterHelp. https://www.betterhelp.com/advice/how-to/how-to-boost-energy-levels-through-the-mind-body-connection/

102.   Team, T. (2025, February 13). How Mindfulness Influences your Design Thinking. Timely.com; Timely Blog. https://www.timely.com/blog/how-mindfulness-influences-your-design-thinking

103.   The Benefits Of Mindfulness Practices For Dementia Patients (2022). Assuredassistedliving.com. https://www.assuredassistedliving.com/the-benefits-of-mindfulness-practices-for-dementia-patients

104.   The Power of a Holistic Approach to Aging. (2024). Humancareny.com. https://www.humancareny.com/blog/holistic-approach-to-aging

105.   The Power of Mindfulness: Easing Arthritis Pain and Improving Well Being. (2023) Arthritis Queensland. https://www.arthritis.org.au/arthritis/arthritis-insights/positive-health-habits/the-power-of-mindfulness-easing-arthritis-pain-and-improving-well-being/

106.   Themelis, K., & Tang, N. K. Y. (2023, January 1). The Management of Chronic Pain: Re-Centring Person-Centred Care. Journal of Clinical Medicine. https://doi.org/10.3390/jcm12226957

107.   Toussaint, L., Nguyen, Q. A., Roettger, C., Dixon, K., Offenbächer, M., Kohls, N., Hirsch, J., & Sirois, F. (2021). Effectiveness of Progressive Muscle Relaxation, Deep Breathing, and Guided Imagery in Promoting Psychological and Physiological States of Relaxation (R. Taylor-Piliae, Ed.). Evidence-Based Complementary and Alternative Medicine. https://doi.org/10.1155/2021/5924040

108.   Turner, J. A., Anderson, M. L., Balderson, B. H., Cook, A. J., Sherman, K. J., & Cherkin, D. C. (2016, November). Mindfulness-based stress reduction and cognitive behavioral therapy for chronic low back pain. PAIN. https://doi.org/10.1097/j.pain.0000000000000635

109.   Tylor Bennett. (2024, September 24). Pain Management for Tension Headaches - Eastside Ideal Health Redmond. Eastside Ideal Health Redmond. https://www.eastsideidealhealth.com/pain-management-for-tension-headaches/

110.   Veehof, M. M., Trompetter, H. R., Bohlmeijer, E. T., & Schreurs, K. M. G. (2016, January 2). Acceptance- and mindfulness-based interventions for the treatment of chronic pain: a meta-analytic review. Cognitive Behaviour Therapy. https://doi.org/10.1080/16506073.2015.1098724

111.   Visualization & Guided Imagery for Pain Relief (The Complete Guide) - Pathways. (2020, May 30). Www.pathways.health.

https://www.pathways.health/blog/visualization-guided-imagery-for-pain-relief/

112. Wasson, R. S., Barratt, C., & O'Brien, W. H. (2020, March 5). Effects of Mindfulness-Based Interventions on Self-compassion in Health Care Professionals: a Meta-analysis. Mindfulness. https://doi.org/10.1007/s12671-020-01342-5

113. Watson, T., Walker, O., Cann, R., & Varghese, A. K. (2022, January 31). The benefits of mindfulness in mental healthcare professionals. F1000Research. https://doi.org/10.12688/f1000research.73729.2

114. West, T. N., Zhou, J., Brantley, M. M., Kim, S. L., Brantley, J., Salzberg, S., Cole, S. W., & Fredrickson, B. L. (2022, March 16). Effect of Mindfulness Versus Loving-kindness Training on Leukocyte Gene Expression in Midlife Adults Raised in Low-Socioeconomic Status Households. Mindfulness. https://doi.org/10.1007/s12671-022-01857-z

115. What is the Best Form of Personal Development. (2024). Morningcoach.com. https://www.morningcoach.com/blog/whatisthebestforofpersonaldevelopment

116. What to Put on a Vision Board: Unlock Your Goals with These 10 Inspiring Ideas | AFFiNE. (2025). Affine.pro. https://affine.pro/blog/what-to-put-on-a-vision-board

117. Whitaker, A. (2023, November 9). 10 Simple Ways to Integrate Mindfulness into Your Daily Routine - SIYLI. Siyli.org. https://siyli.org/resources/blog/10-simple-ways-to-integrate-mindfulness-into-your-daily-routine

118.   Wright, K. W. (2023, June 21). Emotional journaling: How to use journaling to process emotions. Day One. https://dayoneapp.com/blog/emotional-journaling/

119.   Yelton, M. J., & Jildeh, T. R. (2023, May 23). Cultural Competence and the Postoperative Experience: Pain Control and Rehabilitation. Arthroscopy, Sports Medicine, and Rehabilitation. https://doi.org/10.1016/j.asmr.2023.04.016

120.   Zeidan, F., & Vago, D. R. (2016, June). Mindfulness meditation-based pain relief: a mechanistic account. Annals of the New York Academy of Sciences. https://doi.org/10.1111/nyas.13153

121.   Zeidan, F., Baumgartner, J. N., & Coghill, R. C. (2019). The neural mechanisms of mindfulness-based pain relief. PAIN Reports. https://doi.org/10.1097/pr9.0000000000000759

122.   Zeidan, F., Grant, J. A., Brown, C. A., McHaffie, J. G., & Coghill, R. C. (2012, June). Mindfulness meditation-related pain relief: Evidence for unique brain mechanisms in the regulation of pain. Neuroscience Letters. https://doi.org/10.1016/j.neulet.2012.03.082

123.   Zhang, D., Lee, E. K. P., Mak, E. C. W., Ho, C. Y., & Wong, S. Y. S. (2021). Mindfulness-based interventions: An overall review. British Medical Bulletin. https://doi.org/10.1093/bmb/ldab005